Tripping
Over the
Truth

The Return of the Metabolic
Theory of Cancer Illuminates a
New and Hopeful Path to a Cure

Travis Christofferson

ISBN: 1500600318
ISBN 13: 9781500600310
Library of Congress Control Number: 2014913140
CreateSpace Independent Publishing Platform
North Charleston, South Carolina

Contents

Acknowledgments

Tom Seyfried, Pete Pedersen, Young Ko, and Dominic D'Agostino – thank you for your extraordinarily generous spirits – and for your grit, creative-vision, passion and tenacity. My wife, when I asked her to read the book, she said, "I don't have to, I lived the book." Thank you for "living" the book with me darling. My shining-star kids, for just being the people you are. That an intrinsic biological program caused atoms from disparate parts of the planet to come together, and sculpt little people capable of wonder, reason, and delightful humor – through such little effort on my part – still befuddles me. My editor, Betty Kelly Sargent, for so adroitly and gently sanding away the rough edges. To my beautiful nieces, my sister-in-law, and Henry, my hilarious nephew. My Parents, I love you. My buddy Joe Pfeiffer for always meeting me at the Independent Ale House after a long day of writing and patiently listening to me babble over a pint.

Both science and non-fiction story telling intrinsically rely on the work of others. It's a building that is continually under construction with scientists knocking out walls, adding rooms, pouring new foundations; while science writers go in and redecorate from time to time. To the builders: Tom Seyfried's *Cancer as a Metabolic Disease*, Pete Pedersen's lifetime of research, Young Ko's tireless efforts, Bert Vogelstein and Charles Swanton's outstanding work, writing, and generosity of time. And to the decorators: Siddhartha Mukherjee for his "masterpiece" The Emperor of All Maladies. More than any other you have established the words that capture the disease of cancer. Robert Bazell for his wonderful book *HER-2*. And Clifton Leaf for both his incredibly insightful book *The Truth in Small Doses*, and for the advice and kind encouragement. You are nothing but class. All of their works I borrowed from heavily. It felt silly re-telling the stories they had already told, especially so considering they were told better than I could ever tell them, but I had to for the natural progression of the book. Thanks to Ilona McClintick for your indispensable advice, and George Yu for "believing in me". Thank you Harrie Verhoeven for allowing me to tell the story of Yvar's courageous fight with cancer. I hope, in the end, it helps to save the lives of others. Everybody at Green's, I love you guys. Thanks to Ed and Lisa Engler, Gay Whalin, and Alisha Butterfield for proofing sections.

Special thanks to Robb Wolf for kicking this whole thing off.

And last, to Brady Christofferson, for being a business partner, an editor, a psychologist, a friend, and a brother.

Dedicated to Blu

The truth of a theory can never be proven; for one never knows if future experience will contradict its conclusions.

-Albert Einstein, 1919

In the Beginning

Few words are as emotionally charged as the word *cancer*. For cancer biologists it is a riddle yet to be solved; a cruel killer and a masterful escape artist. To those it has yet to affect, it is an abstraction, something terrifying but distant. Many have intimate stories attached to the word. Some are stories of triumph, but many are of a struggle with a foe that proves too relentless, too savvy, and too hard to pin down. Still today, perhaps the most terrifying quality of *cancer* is profound helplessness. We all know that if cancer wants to win, it most likely will.

Human history is a story of conquest over the natural world—our triumph over the procuring of food, water, and shelter and combating disease. We figure out ways to not be helpless. Just recently we have gotten very good at it. When we lived in caves and throughout the Bronze and Iron Ages, humans could expect to live into their twenties. The Romans were only able to boost life expectancy to the late twenties. By the early twentieth century, the average life span was up to thirty-one, but between then and now, in only about one hundred years, the average global life expectancy has more than doubled. Today an adult male, born in the West, can expect to live to be about seventy-six and a female to eighty-one. The global average is sixty-seven.

Infectious disease alone conspired to keep life-expectancy abysmally low throughout the majority of our past. When Louis Pasteur showed the world that there were invisible, alien-like microbial life forms lurking all around us and thriving in the inner city filth created by the industrial revolution, it was largely a matter of simply cleaning up. After that came vaccines, and on the heels of vaccines came the miracle of antibiotics, "substances that do deeds transcending all medical preconceptions," as Nobel laureate Peyton Rous so elegantly put it. One by one, we were beating back the forces that prevented us from living out our natural life span.

Our drive to live unencumbered by the shackles of nature is so relentless that even our natural life span is now on the table. Scientist Leonard Hayflick described aging as "an artifact of civilization," opening the door to the possibility that aging is not the inevitable process it was always thought to be. It might be malleable, delayed, or switched off entirely. This enticing possibility has put aging in the cross hairs of an imaginative new sect of molecular biologists who see no limit to what can be achieved. Mankind's unique desire to live forever, to discover a fountain of youth, is now said to be within reach. It is only a matter of time. Ethical and moral issues aside, there is nothing mystical about this. It is just an engineering project like going to the moon. It *really is* just a matter of time. Stem cells, those wondrous propagators of youth, will be manipulated into forming tissues or even entire organs, replacing our parts as they wear out. Genes will be tweaked, turned on, and turned off, unfolding an intrinsic program of eternal youth. Even Google is in on the dream. Recently they announced a venture called California Life Company (CALICO), and its stated goal is to employ the power of supercomputing to "fight aging and solve death."

The uncomfortable truth of cancer threatens our exalted march toward immortality. Cancer stands alone as our most ardent, confusing, shapeshifting, and devastating enemy. The numbers don't lie. This year, almost six hundred thousand Americans will die from cancer. One in two men and one in three women will be diagnosed in their lifetimes. Despite embellished announcements from government actuaries, the real death rates from cancer are the same today as they were in the 1950s. We can't seem to penetrate its elusive armor, and it's not for lack of trying. Cancer receives more funding from the National Institutes of Health (NIH) than any other disease. Not to mention that it is under investigation at every major pharmaceutical company around the world.

This book is the result of my journey to discover why cures for cancer have remained so elusive. Why in a century of breathtaking progress where the word *immortality* is actually taken seriously, has progress in treating cancer remained so static? Radiation, still one of the main methods of treatment, was invented well over one hundred years ago when horses and buggies occupied the streets.

There is no shortage of ideas for the stagnant progress. Some suggest that because of the collective failure of academia, government, and industry, a culture has developed that discourages risk taking and encourages narrow thinking. Some say it is simply due to not enough funding. Others believe that it is a manifestation of the complexity of the disease itself. Cancer is just that difficult.

I've tried to look for the answer to this question in a place others haven't—one protected by an invisible dome of dogma, large-scale group think, and institutional inertia. Maybe the reason for the stunted progress goes far deeper than we thought. Maybe it is fundamental, going all the way to the scientific bedrock at the true heart of the disease. Could it be a reason that exists in the guts of the science itself? To utter it is heretical, to say it out loud invites scoffs, dismissal, even outright anger, but here it is. Maybe we've mischaracterized the origin of cancer. Maybe cancer is not a genetic disease after all. Maybe we are losing the war against cancer because scientists are chasing a flawed scientific paradigm, and cancer is not a disease of damaged DNA but rather one of defective metabolism.

In the Beginning

This idea didn't start with me. I stumbled onto it a few years ago when I was introduced to the idea in a book called *Cancer as a Metabolic Disease*. Its author, Thomas Seyfried, PhD, of Boston College, is bold, confident, outspoken, and very smart. The idea that cancer was metabolic did not come from Seyfried either. The original claim came from a remarkable German scientist named Otto Warburg in 1924. Throughout the century Warburg's claim was a side note in reviews on the subject of cancer. It never really gained a critical mass of supporters. It remained just a curious observation. By the 1960's, his theory had all but faded into oblivion. When he died in 1970, his antiquated hypothesis could have died with him, but ideas can live on and, as in Warburg's case, can even be resuscitated. It would have slipped into oblivion if Peter ("Pete") Pedersen of Johns Hopkins University School of Medicine hadn't noticed it and methodically nurtured it back to life. In the 1970s and 1980s, he was alone in his belief that Warburg was right.

Warburg's observation was this: cancer cells have a perverted method of generating energy. They truncate the conversion of glucose (sugar) into energy. They depend much less on the efficient process of respiratory energy creation, using oxygen—instead relying much more on the ancient and highly inefficient pathway known as fermentation. Later in his career, Warburg contended that this was the true origin of cancer. The cell's ability to generate energy through the oxidative pathway is damaged, and the cell reverts to fermentation. He said, "Cancer, above all other diseases, has countless secondary causes. But, even for cancer, there is only one prime cause. Summarized in a few words, the prime cause of cancer is the replacement of the respiration of oxygen in normal body cells by a fermentation of sugar."

In the summer of 2012, Seyfried released his book, and his ideas to the world. Expanding upon Warburg's hypothesis (and Pedersen's work, following Warburg's death), Seyfried noted that across the board, cancer cells have damage to a cellular organelle called a *mitochondrion* or, if more than one, *mitochondria*. Typically each animal cell, including those of humans, has one thousand to two thousand mitochondria. Mitochondria are thought of as the cellular power plants. They generate energy through oxidative respiration, supplying the body with the energy it needs to function (later pages will show how mitochondria are damaged in the first place). The damaged mitochondria, unable to generate enough energy for cellular survival, then send out emergency signals to the nucleus, a 911 call pleading for it to switch on emergency generators. Once this call is made and DNA responds, the entire complexion of the cell changes. It begins to exhibit the hallmark features of cancer: uncontrolled proliferation, genomic instability (the increased probability that DNA mutation will occur), evasion of cell death, and so forth. The process is probably an ancient mechanism designed to nurture cells through transient moments when little oxygen was available that undoubtedly occurred as the planet's first cells evolved toward increasing complexity—a primordial survival mechanism, a vestige of our evolutionary past. The bottom line is this: damage to mitochondria happens first, then genomic instability, and then mutations to DNA. The upshot, according to Seyfried, is that the mutations to DNA, thought to precipitate and drive the disease, are only a side effect, sending researchers on a multidecade, multibillion-dollar wild goose chase. It is a bold proclamation, and the majority of cancer researchers disagree with Seyfried's assertions, but history is replete with examples of humanity getting big issues wrong for extended periods of time.

Like Dr. Barry Marshall, labeled a quack by the medical community for his claim that an unknown species of bacteria caused ulcers rather than stress, the accepted but ambiguous perpetrator. According to medical convention, bacteria couldn't exist in the acidic environment of the stomach. Undeterred, once Marshall was convinced that he had isolated the elusive bacterium, he then grew it until he had a flask brimming with murky liquid that housed billions of bacterial cells. Then, in an act of desperation, he did what he felt was the only option to prove his claim: he drank the liquid. The highly publicized ulcer that erupted in his stomach was documented in a medical journal, unequivocally proving to the establishment that the bacterium (identified as *helicobacter pylori*) could, by itself, cause ulcers. Once ridiculed for his outlandish proclamation, Marshall was awarded a Nobel Prize.

Of course the vast majority of cancer biologists still believe that the origin of cancer has been conclusively decided and the chapter is closed. I intend to show how a single experiment in 1976 merged several lines of evidence into a grand unified theory that cancer originated from mutations to DNA. The theory, called the somatic mutation theory (SMT) of cancer, was accepted conclusively. There was a worldwide eureka moment. There were cheers and backslapping. Nobel Prizes were given. The war was waged with a new sense of resolve. It was not a bold leap of imagination to envision a smart war from there, one that used drugs "targeted" to the products of oncogenes (cancer-causing genes), honing in on cancer cells and sparing normal cells. The days of toxic chemotherapy and radiation would soon be relics of an era of medieval medicine akin to bloodletting and leeches.

Any scientist will tell you that theories are anything but permanent. It is a mistake to be seduced into believing that textbooks alone provide validation of a scientific theory. Theories are ephemeral things. They are only our closest approximation of the truth at a fleeting moment in an otherwise infinite continuum of discovery. Look at the cycle of succession that physics has experienced in its quest to describe the universe over the last three hundred years. Newton's classic mechanics established the laws of the universe in 1687. That is until Einstein's theory of relativity replaced it in 1915, once and for all providing us with a definitive description of the universe. But even Einstein's elegant and once undisputed theory is now being chipped away as the cryptic and arcane string theory takes form.

Could Warburg have been right? At this strange junction only one thing is certain. Our understanding of cancer is still in its infancy.

When I completed my undergraduate degree at Montana State University, I believed what the textbooks said—after all, the SMT of cancer was well established, lifetimes of careful thinking and solid research backed it, or so I had been told. Like everybody, I wondered why progress in treating cancer seemed so slow. It seemed like breakthroughs were perpetually "around the corner" but never materialized. When I stumbled onto Seyfried's book during my last year of graduate school, it was certainly enlightening. If true, it explained the profound lack of progress in combating the disease. I was not entirely convinced but intrigued enough to keep looking. That's when I looked more extensively at the latest incarnation of the government's war against cancer: a massive, multinational project funded by the National Cancer Institute (NCI) called The Cancer Genome Atlas (TCGA) that began in 2006.

Most researchers, especially those at the head of the NCI, unwaveringly believe that cancer is caused by DNA mutations that are thought to sequentially rewire critical cellular circuitry – marching a cell, step by step, toward becoming a chaotic, aggressive, uncontrolled, and invasive killer. So in order to understand cancer in its entirety, the entire genome of a cancer cell (all the DNA inside the cell) would have to be sequenced identifying and cataloging all the "driver" mutations within the DNA. This is the goal of the TCGA. It is The Manhattan Project of cancer, an outcome-based effort supposed to be the final chapter in the war against cancer. Laboratories throughout the world are churning out the genomic sequence of multiple types of cancer with inconceivable speed and efficiency.

In the Beginning

The project compares the sequence of normal DNA to that of different cancer types to determine the exact mutations responsible for the origin and progression of the malignancies. Researchers will finally know cancer in its entirety—they will be staring the shape-shifting enemy directly in the face. Make no mistake, everything has led to this—If one could fast forward through one hundred years of research, every intellectual avenue would lead to TCGA as the flag-ship endeavor required for a cure. That is *if* cancer is really precipitated and driven by mutations to DNA.

When I dug into the data coming out of TCGA, what I found was stunning. Nothing made sense. Prior to the project, researchers largely believed the sequencing data would reveal an orderly sequence of maybe three to eight genes that when mutated, manifested in a specific type of cancer—an identifying signature like a fingerprint—and they would work off this mutational signature with cures to follow. But what the sequence data revealed was anything but orderly. It exposed an almost random collection of mutations—not a single one, or any combination for that matter, being absolutely responsible for initiating the disease. For the SMT to work, mutational patterns had to be found that explained the origin of a given type of cancer. The cause had to precede and explain the effect. Critically, the mutations determined to start and drive the disease were different from person to person, vastly different. No single mutation or no combination of mutations could be identified that were absolutely required for the disease to start. Other than a few commonly mutated oncogenes, the mutational pattern appeared largely random.

Beyond the hype of the media and pharmaceutical companies, hidden deep in the scientific journals, the scientists are interpreting the data streaming out of TCGA, and their words give us a far different picture: "immense therapeutic implications," "sobering realization," and "incredibly complex." The prominent University of Southern

California oncologist Dr. David Agus (who treated Steve Jobs), simmering with frustration in a recent speech, even suggested that we stop trying to understand the disease altogether and just throw darts at it, hoping to find therapies that work.

This is when the story became really interesting. In the fall of 2012, I began to call and e-mail the scientists involved in the project. I wanted to know if they saw what I saw or if I had misinterpreted the data or was missing something. What I found was a collective moment of shock and confusion. Some acknowledged the stunning randomness, capitulating to the complexity of the disease, declared their resignation—"Maybe it is just too hard to figure out." Others had begun to modify the SMT in order for it to continue to make sense. Some, like Pedersen and Seyfried, had already moved on. To be sure, on the whole, the cancer community was confused and reorganizing.

The success rate of the drugs designed to target the mutations identified by TCGA is abysmal. More than seven hundred have been developed, and only one, GLEEVEC, has made a meaningful difference in the lives of cancer patients. Most "targeted" drugs might give a cancer patient a few more months. Some offer no survival benefit at all and can cost more than $100,000 for a course of treatment. When it comes to oncological drugs, a relationship between price and value doesn't exist. The FDA has set the bar low for approval, requiring only that a new drug shrink a tumor, without considering the ultimate arbiter of success: survival. As a consequence, these drugs get approved. Call it what you will, but to charge a patient a fortune for zero benefit is immoral. GLEEVEC was hailed as a "proof of principle" that targeting drugs to mutations was the right approach. But in all probability, GLEEVEC exerts its efficacy by altering pathways turned on by damaged metabolism—perhaps by hanging up the 911 call alluded to earlier.

Why have the promised targeted drugs failed to materialize? First TCGA failed to identify the mutations that definitively caused any given type of cancer. As a consequence, researchers have not been able to find the right target or targets. Second, another ominous discovery came from TCGA, one that cast a dark cloud over the hope for any meaningful breakthroughs anytime soon. From a genetic perspective, drug design is a brutally difficult game of "catch me if you can." The mutational targets are not only vastly different from person to person, but they can even vary spectacularly from cell to cell within the same tumor, leaving pharmaceutical chemists with an impossibly difficult task. Followed to its conclusion, the SMT of cancer placed the outcome of many cases locked in the jaws of inevitability.

The therapeutic implications of the metabolic theory are that every type of cancer is treatable, because every type of cancer has the same beautiful, metabolic target painted on its back, regardless of the tissue of origin or type of cancer. Rather than targeting mutations that were here one second gone the next, the metabolic theory put researchers back in the driver's seat. It put cancer back in the realm of curable, implying that we were not helpless against the disease. It restored hope.

Although unknown and underappreciated, the therapies derived from the logic that cancer stems from damaged metabolism have shown remarkable results. Metabolic therapies flow from a simple framework of logic. Every cancer cell has the same defect and the same exploitable target. (I will explore the promising metabolic therapies developed to date and nontoxic approaches that exploit the metabolic intransigence of the cancer cell.) A cancer drug discovered by Dr. Young Hee Ko in Pedersen's lab at Johns Hopkins in 2000 that acts like a heat-seeking missile attacking the target Warburg put a "red dot" on almost a century ago, but sadly, it was hung up in a heated court battle.

A dietary protocol developed by Seyfried that has shown promise to slow the growth of cancer and work synergistically with existing therapies while mitigating side effects. Although unquestionably in their infancy, metabolic therapies have demonstrated incredible promise. Without question they merit more attention. My hope is that this book will cause that to happen.

Few things ignite passion like questioning an entrenched paradigm, especially such an emotionally charged one that affects so many people. I learned this in 2013 after writing an article titled, "It Is Biology's Most Fundamental Question: What Is the Origin of Cancer?" It was posted on the blog of the Paleo Diet advocate, Robb Wolf, and linked to Twitter and Facebook by Wolf's good friend, Tim Ferriss. Both Wolf and Ferriss are *New York Times* bestselling authors, and sort of a GenX version of the Renaissance man, both have huge followings. After writing the article, I had difficulty finding a home for it. Nobody knew who I was, and nobody was willing to take a chance and publish it. But Wolf and Ferriss are different, they are idea driven. They embrace outside-the-box thinking and risk taking.

This is the e-mail that Wolf sent to Ferriss:

Tim! Hey, hope all is well. This is an article written by a grad student studying the work of one of my favorite researchers...talking about a non-genetic basis for the development of some (possibly many) cancers. So, I REALLY want to run this on my blog...it is fucking gold content. BUT...you have way more bandwidth than I do and this stuff can, will, save lives. It deserves the largest messaging we can muster IMO. I've attached an interview I did with Thomas Seyfried (researcher at Boston College) that I did nearly 10 years ago, also one of his papers on ketogenic diet and brain cancer. My business side says "run it yourself!" My hippy-save-the-world side knows you could affect way more change with this, if it's something you are interested in running. Hope all is well with you, let me know what you think.

In the Beginning

Once the article was posted the comments poured in. Challenging dogmatic concepts tends to galvanize people. Some are naturally, almost intrinsically wired to embrace new or different ideas, others are the exact opposite, dismissing them at the first sentence. One thing both sides have in common is an almost instantaneous gut-reaction in one direction or the other, a reaction that usually has little to do with the actual evidence.

The article was like a match that ignited a flame. There was so much more to this story. For me this was just the beginning. It was a scientific detective story that had to be told and it became the focus of my life for the next two years. Soon it became apparent, in interview after interview, that the story went far beyond the cold, empirical data, it tapped into base psychology, human limitations, economic incentives, and the deep-rooted, powerful force of groupthink, forces that carry the inertia of the Titanic. Scientific progress doesn't glide from one exalted epiphany to the next, like the story of Isaac Newton getting hit on his head by an apple. It is a torch carried by human beings, it lurches, stumbles, wanders into dead ends, and then finds its way back out. It doesn't march in a straight line – it trips its way toward the truth. But the beautiful thing about science is that no matter how bumpy the ride, eventually, because of the process itself, the truth is slowly, inevitably, mapped out.

This book is a culmination of that scientific pilgrimage. It is both the scientific and human story of the revival of Warburg's old theory and the profound therapeutic consequences that travel with it. It is a look into the continuing quest to discover the nature of cancer from a different angle, taking all the puzzle pieces and assembling them in a new way.

This book is about the continuing quest to discover the true origin of cancer, reduce the problem to its core elements, define it in its simplest terms, and find the critical molecular events that manifest in uncontrolled proliferation. As veteran cancer researcher Bert Vogelstein has said many times, "Make no mistake—we are not there yet." Agus said we shouldn't even try to understand the disease, it is just too hard. Others have said the same thing. We should learn to treat it without understanding it. The question is worth asking: why should we try? Why is it so important? Because to cure cancer, we first have to know it. If we've learned one thing from the battles we've fought against disease, it is that progress does not happen without understanding.

This is one story, one version of humanity's continuous struggle to uncover the origin of cancer—one of the most important struggles we still face. This is a story of discovery and hope.

Part 1

How Cancer Became Known as a Genetic Disease

During a career devoted entirely to research and extending over 60 years, he made an exceptionally large number of highly origi-nal and far-reaching contributions to cell biology and biochem-istry. Lewis and Randall, [in] the preface to 'Thermodynamics and the free energy of chemical substances', liken the edifice of science to a cathedral built by the efforts of a few architects and many workers, In this sense Warburg was one of the small band of real architects of his generation.
—Hans Krebs, author of Otto Warburg: Cell Physiologist, Biochemist, and Eccentric

Chimney Boys

As Percivall Pott walked the London streets, he could only guess at the brand of manure he was stepping in. It could be cow, goat, horse, or any combination. He covered his mouth. The smells were horrifying, especially considering that it was thought that pestilence traveled through smell. It was 1775, and it would be almost a century before Pasteur eased people's anxiety and assigned microorganisms as the culprit, not smell.

Pott didn't have to be there. As a surgeon, he was largely separated from the squalor of the masses that exploded into London as the Industrial Revolution took hold. He was there because of a nagging question that wouldn't leave him alone. In the dim light he saw people piled in shacks, ten to a single room, sleeping on sawdust to shield them from the damp dirt floor. The sounds of babies crying pierced the air.

A girl emerged from one of the shacks, pulled out a match, and lit a street lantern. In the years to come, a match factory would emerge not far away and employ almost exclusively girls like her. White phosphorous would be used in the process, and the fumes of the corrosive chemical would find their way into the girls, causing a condition called *phossy jaw.* It began as a toothache. Soon the whole jaw ached and began to rot, emitting the necrotic smell of decay. Doctors would diagnose the condition by putting the girls into a dark room where the affected bones would glow a greenish-white color. Surgeons like Pott could save the girls only by removing the affected bones quickly, or organ failure and death would rapidly follow.

From another shanty, Pott heard the sound of a convulsing, consumptive cough. He was intimately familiar with the sound—it meant tuberculosis. Almost everybody in inner city London had it. Pott's most important work was with tuberculosis. He described the migrating path that TB could sometimes follow into the spine, resulting in loss of limb function. His description became definitive, and the illness came to be known as Pott's Disease. But this night he was here for a different reason.

As the smoke stacks transformed the landscape of London into a faceless, apathetic, churning economic juggernaut, young boys were often indentured to sweep chimneys, and Pott noticed a sharp rise in a curious condition that afflicted them. They came in complaining of painful "warts" on their scrotums. Even though they appeared to be a rare form of cancerous growth, other doctors wrote off the "soot warts" as syphilis. But Pott couldn't reconcile this diagnosis with the fact the condition seemed to overwhelmingly afflict chimney boys. A venereal disease like syphilis would spread evenly among everyone, not preferentially by occupation. Something about the condition had to correlate with the occupation.

This was why Pott found himself walking through the slums at night. Earlier in the day, one of the boys had come to him, complaining of scrotal pain. When Pott examined him, he found the typical open, festering sores. The boy said he lived on this street with other chimney boys, and Pott wanted to see for himself how they lived. He had a hypothesis that he couldn't get out of his mind. Could the constant grime and soot that the boys were in contact with be the cause of their affliction?

Conditions during the Industrial Revolution were so harsh that newborns had a coin flip's chance of living to age five. If they did, that was when they began to work, often fourteen-hour days, six days a week. They could look forward to this severely spartan existence until about age thirty-five, which was the life expectancy for a Londoner of the time. Even among this harsh backdrop, the chimney boys stood out. The boys, usually orphans, were cast into indentured servitude under the label of "apprentice" to master sweeps. Stripped down and covered in oil, the boys were told to climb up inside the chimneys and rid them of the black soot and ash. The disposable castaways of society scrubbed the fallout of economic advancement. They were viewed as filthy, consumptive misfits, and people took wide paths around them on the streets.

Pott stopped when he saw the shanty next to the tavern the boy had described. Muffled sounds of patrons emanated from inside as working men shared a beer in a fleeting moment of respite from the drudgery of their existence. The wet slop belched under his feet as he walked to the side of the street where light from a lamp barely illuminated the inside of the shanty. There were roughly a dozen boys inside almost piled on top of one another. He walked closer, it was as he suspected. The chimney sweeps were still coated in the oil and grime that covered them during the day. They didn't or weren't able to clean themselves at night. This anchored his theory that the soot was causing cancer.

Pott walked home, the theory solidifying as the sounds and smells of the fitful London night faded behind him. Under the light of his lamp, he worked late into the night, documenting his theory and establishing that the cause of the epidemic was "a lodgment of soot in the rugae of the scrotum." What Pott established was a breakthrough in the history of cancer, the first documentation of an external agent as the cause of cancer. Today we know these agents as carcinogens. It was an observation that would forever be synonymous with the disease.

The fact that an external agent could cause cancer changed the way doctors thought about the disease. Cancer was merged with the environment. Doctors could look suspiciously at environmental suspects lurking around us, somehow transforming the body into a fit of uncontrolled growth. Pott's observation turned into a growing list of suspects, and a theory emerged from the list. It was clear that carcinogens were altering the cell and mutating a critical component that was responsible for controlling cellular division. Although the mutated component was unknown, cause and effect were established. A line was drawn from carcinogen to cancer. The theory would eventually become known as the somatic mutation theory of cancer. At the very least, large gaps of understanding aside, Pott's observation led doctors to the idea of prevention. Even though mass efforts to that end would take decades of slow moving social change, at least we were getting to know the enemy, at least we weren't entirely helpless.

Chaotic Chromosomes

Rudolf Virchow, born in 1821, was considered the "father of modern pathology." With his microscope, he was able to recognize the fundamental pathology of cancer: uncontrolled growth. An uninhibited hyper drive of cellular division that physically damaged surrounding tissues, hijacked nutrients and space, degraded confining membranes, then traveling through blood vessels to other sites to again corrupt and steal from healthy tissue, in all a parasite emerging from the body itself. He identified the *how* of cancer's assault on the body, but he could only guess as to the *why*.

An outspoken and opinionated man, he refused to hold his tongue on a variety of subjects, many political, which often landed him in trouble. Prussian Minister Otto von Bismarck was so annoyed by Virchow's antagonism that he once challenged him to a duel, but Virchow declined, stating that it was an uncivilized way to settle a dispute. Despite his views, Virchow's skill in pathology seemed to trump his antagonist personality and return him to favor. His empirical style was in sharp contrast to the times when disease was described as the arcane imbalance of "humors," a supernatural description that had dominated medicine for centuries. He refused to entertain any cause of a disease other than ones stemming from variables that could be seen, touched, or measured. He pulled disease from the realm of the mystical into the tangible where real treatment was possible. He may have described how cancer acted, but it was his student, David Paul von Hansemann, that made the conceptual leap to the apparent *why* of cancer. The leap would plant the seed of the modern version of the SMT of cancer.

How Cancer Became Known as a Genetic Disease

Hansemann was born in to a prominent German family in 1858. His Uncle Adolf, on his father's side, took up where his grandfather left off, continuing the family's rise to prominence in business and politics. Adolf landed in banking and helped to finance the critical railway expansion across Germany, eventually even financing Germany's expenses during the Danish and Franco-Prussian Wars.

Adolf's little brother (David's father), Gustav, was not as successful in business. He managed a woolen factory without much enthusiasm, realizing that his interests lay outside the family traditions, he turned to an academic career in physics and mathematics. He wrote three books, exposing a whimsical imagination and a creative way of observing the world around him, traits he passed onto his son, David Paul.

As a young man, Hansemann was accepted into the German medical school system, which was regarded as the best in the world. The original staff of Johns Hopkins and the Mayo brothers were undergoing training in Germany at the time, learning cutting-edge techniques as they established their respective institutions. Like his father, Hansemann excelled in the German system. After compulsory military service, he settled in to study pathology under Virchow. He knew that Virchow had established that cancer was a pathological growth, but Hansemann wanted to know why. Luck intervened.

In the nearby city of Prague, a scientist named Walther Fleming was playing around with a blue dye that stained certain cellular components but not others, allowing for contrast. The dye made it possible to visualize cellular structure. The components the dye did stain were threadlike objects that elegantly lined up in the center of the cell right before cellular division took place, like school children told to form a line. Fleming had no idea what these objects were, so he coined the term *chromosomes* (colored bodies).

Hansemann heard about Fleming's work with the dye and wanted to try it on cancer cells. He noticed something striking. Rather than the symmetry and order that Fleming observed, the chromosomes of cancer cells were in complete chaos. They were bent, broken, and duplicated. Rather than children lining up neatly, they looked like kids at play. The imaginative propensity Hansemann inherited from his father then took over. In an inspired conceptual leap, he assigned cancer's pathological growth to the chromosomal chaos, reasoning that the chaotic chromosomes must be the *why* that his mentor Virchow had missed. Hansemann assigned the pathogenesis of cancer to asymmetric mitoses. As he described it, "the conversion of normal cells to cancerous ones involves the acquisition of intracellular-arising abnormalities to their hereditary material."

In addition to his proposal that chromosomes were responsible for cancer's uncontrolled growth, he coined the terms *anaplasia* and *dedifferentiation*. Both described the qualitative path that the tumor cells traveled from a state of differentiation to a state of less differentiation, as if the cell was traveling in reverse. Differentiation described the final tissue type of a cell. For example, during the developmental process, a stem cell would differentiate into a liver cell, thus allowing for the tissue level of specialization. The fact that Hansemann was able to establish this as a dominant feature of cancer in 1890 was remarkable. Even today, the loss of differentiation (anaplasia) is considered one of the most important aspects of cancer. Cancer cells could wildly undulate from a state of dedifferentiation and back, which explained why some tumors contained multiple tissue types. Teeth and hair follicles had even been found inside tumors.

As part of his theoretical framework, Hansemann insisted that any theory describing cancer must have "Gesamtheit," meaning that it must describe clinical behavior in the patient as well as the pathology, epidemiology, and etiological characteristics of tumors. Hansemann's philosophical arc continued, and he wrote a book translated as *The Philosophy of Cancer*, which earned him ridicule from colleagues.

He soon returned to the more empirical side of the disease, applying his theory of anaplasia to the practical problem of diagnosis and the nomenclature of tumors, sparking modern histopathology.

Pott had connected external agents to cancer, but Hansemann's observation was internal—a structural defect that contrasted normal cells from cancer cells. It took a short leap of imagination to stitch the external causes Pott discovered to the internal abnormalities that Hansemann observed. The theory linking carcinogens to damaged chromosomes became known as the SMT. If doctors thought the groundwork of the theory was laid with only the gaps to be filled in, they were in for a surprising twist, a discovery that would shake the foundation of cancer biology, changing its course for the better part of a century.

Is Cancer Infectious?

The first thing Peyton Rous thought of was his mother. It was 1902, and he was in his second year of medical school at Johns Hopkins in Baltimore. He knew how much she had given up for him. After his father's death, instead of returning to her large, wealthy family in Texas, she chose to stay in Baltimore so that he could get the best education possible.

"Is it bleeding?" he asked his anatomy partner in an anxious whisper.

His head cocked sideways to peer at Rous's finger, he said, "Yes, it's bleeding."

Rous looked at the tuberculosis-riddled bone he had just cut his hand on. He was doing an autopsy on a patient who had died from TB, and the bones were still saturated with the infectious microbe. A pit formed in Rous's stomach. He would have to wait and see if the patented tube corpuse formed, a pathological structure that provided definitive evidence of a localized tuberculosis infection. If it didn't, he was in the clear. If it did...

He knew what the pathologist would say. He had seen the pictures in his textbook. He could feel the infection slowly working its way up his arm, and the lymph nodes closest to the infected finger were beginning to swell.

As he rolled the tissue of Rous's arm between his finger and thumb, the doctor said, "It appears you've been infected." It still stung to hear it, and whatever hope lingered was gone. "I would recommend removing the auxiliary nodes, and then, well...then there is...no more can be done other than for you to go away and get well."

That hadn't crossed his mind. Of course a leave would be recommended.

The surgery went well, and the surgeon told Rous that he should recover fully. He looked down at his bandaged arm. He had sent a letter to his uncle in Texas, explaining what had happened. He extending his desire to come to his ranch in Texas to convalesce for the year that the university advised. If he kept his health and the infection did not spread, he would work to earn his keep.

When he saw the postman arrive, he hoped that a response from his uncle would be there. It was. He anxiously tore open the envelope and stopped after the first line, "We would be happy to have you, nephew." His bags were already packed.

When he arrived in Texas, Rous was struck by the sharp contrast between the stuffy, intellectual atmosphere of his prestigious East Coast university and the laid-back Texas ranch culture. Work was hard, and the days could be long, but the camaraderie and peace of wide open spaces captivated him. It had been three months since his accident, and he was feeling fine. One day as he walked through the town adjacent to the ranch, he noticed a friend of the family standing on the stoop of the saloon. Rous went to say hello. As they talked, the friend invited Rous to join him and his ranch hands on a cattle drive that would began in few days and would last about three months. The idea intrigued him, maybe because it was so far removed from his other life. He welcomed the idea of living on the open range and sleeping under the stars.

The next three months left an impression on Rous like no other, and they shaped his thinking for the rest of his life. The cattle drive was filled with days of singular purpose. It was pure in its simplicity: riding horseback, working with others through hand signals and gesture alone, and feeling the companionship. He was a guest, yet the ranch hands treated him like a brother. They relied on each other. He slept on the ground under the stars with them. He was able to find meaning where others would find routine. Those months, when he earned the respect and shared the solidarity of the simple but generous cowboys, left a profound impression on him that he would later say he "drew comfort from the rest of his life."

Because of his cattle drive experience, Rous found meaning where others didn't. Seven years later, when a woman walked into the Rockefeller Institute in New York City carrying a Plymouth Rock hen with a large tumor on its breast, others may have scoffed and sent her away. She wasn't versed in the language of science, but something was strange about this chicken and the disease that it carried, and she was astute enough to recognize that it was worth further study.

Rous didn't dismiss her concerns; he embraced them. Maybe she was on to something. Like Pott and Hansemann, the progression in the understanding of cancer was punctuated by the few who could see where others could not, the few who had transcendent moments of imagination that connected points of light into a single image.

Operating on a hunch the first thing he did was to see if the cancer was transmittable. He surgically removed the tumor, sliced it into tiny bits, and thrust the bits into the breast and peritoneal cavity of two young hens. A month later, one of the young hens developed a mass where the tumor was transplanted. It was the same spindle cell sarcoma that had afflicted the first hen. Rous repeated the process with the young hen, removing the tumor and transplanting pieces of it into other young hens. He wrote, "In this paper is reported the first avian tumor that has proved transplantable to other individuals. It is a spindle-celled sarcoma of a hen, which has thus far has been propagated to the fourth generation." The fact that the tumor proved to be transmittable raised another question: what from the original tumor caused the cancer to be transmittable? It could be as simple as the transferred live cancer cells continuing their propagation within a new host. The problem had to be further reduced.

To illuminate the first issue, Rous filtered out the cancer cells from a tumor sample, leaving a liquid. The filter he used filtered out bacterial cells but allowed another known infectious agent to pass: a virus. If the filtered tumor material could induce cancer in another chicken, he reasoned, the cancer had to be transmitted virally. After injecting a new chicken with his filtered tumor material, he waited. When Rous saw what was unmistakably cancer growing in the newly infected chicken he knew that he had changed the paradigm of cancer forever. This was the first proven viral cause for a solid tumor.

Just as important as Rous proving that a virus could cause a solid tumor was the context his discovery fell into. From the early 1860s, when Pasteur proved that microorganisms caused disease, humanity's worst blights stemmed from infection. Cholera, typhus, typhoid fever, TB, and the plague were all caused by invisible invaders that people were helpless against. When Rous made his discovery, polio, the viral disease that crippled both children and adults, was raging in waves of epidemics across Europe and America. It struck in the summer months, leaving thousands paralyzed or crippled in its wake. The discovery that yet another affliction was caused by an infectious microorganism fit seamlessly into what was known and believed.

The idea that cancer could be viral moved effortlessly into the imaginations of cancer researchers and ignited a media firestorm. After Rous published a paper describing his discovery, the *New York Times* ran an article titled "Is Cancer Infectious?" Researchers were confronted with the question of how cancer could be caused by both Pott's carcinogens and Rous's virus. Presented with separate causes—external carcinogens and internal infection—it seemed probable that both causes were converging to the same alteration in the cell, but where? How could a virus and environmental agents both manifest the same disease? The broken chromosomes Hansemann observed became the top suspect. Rous's cancer virus was a thorn in the side of cancer biology. It flew in the face of the SMT of cancer, breaking it apart at the seams. The discovery that viruses could cause cancer would prevent the formation of a single, comprehensive theory on the origin of cancer for most of the twentieth century.

Warburg's War

Otto Warburg found himself in a pensive mood. Behind him, the clanking sounds of metal hitting metal rang from the mess tent as the cooks prepared food. He looked out at the barren, gray landscape, flattened by the incessant, cold Russian wind. The same wind was slapping at his face.

It was 1918, and Warburg thought about what he had seen. The front lines of World War I had an atmosphere of suffering unlike any other. A war of attrition meant that bodies piled up. The transient stalemates were broken by waves of attacks or, worse, by slow-moving, indiscriminate clouds of newly created war gases. It was the fourth year of the war, and as if the degree of misery cast upon the world's youth was not enough, Mother Nature threw in her own in the form of an influenza virus the likes of which had never been seen and has never been seen since. The blanket of pestilence started in Spain and circled the globe. When it disappeared, the body count was appalling. Nine million were killed in battle, but forty million died from influenza. The scale of suffering was staggering.

Warburg was not there because he had to be. He had volunteered. His family, friends, and colleagues told him that his place was not participating in one of humanity's most horrific wars. It was at home in the laboratory.

"Warburg!"

He turned to see who had shouted his name. Under a canopy, a soldier was sorting letters and calling out names.

"This one is for you," the soldier said as he held out a letter.

Much was swirling around in his mind as he opened the letter and began to read.

Dear Colleague,

You will be surprised to receive a letter from me because up to now we have walked around each other, without actually getting to know each other. I even fear that by this letter I might arouse something like displeasure; but I *must* write.

I gather that you are one of the most able and most promising younger physiologists in Germany and that the representation of your special subject here is rather mediocre. I also gather that you are on active service in a very dangerous position so that your life continuously hangs on a thread: now for a moment please slip out of your skin and into that of another clear-eyed being and ask yourself: Is this not madness? Can your place out there not be taken by any average man; is it not important to prevent the loss of valuable men in that bloody struggle. You know this well and must agree with me. Yesterday I spoke to Professor Kraus who entirely shares my opinion and is also willing to make arrangements for you to be claimed for other work.

I therefore entreat you, as a consequence of what I have said, that you may assist us in our endeavors to safeguard your life. I beg you to send me, after a few hours of serious heart-searching, a few lines so that we may know here that our efforts will not fail on account of *your* attitude.

In the anxious hope that in this matter, as an exception, reason will for once prevail, I am with cordial greetings,

Yours sincerely,
Albert Einstein

He thought back to his childhood home and being greeted by his charming, witty mother, traits that he liked to imagine shaped some of his better aspects. His mind wandered to his father, his touchstone, who occupied the most prestigious physics position in Imperial Germany, the physics chair at the University of Berlin. But Otto's ambition laid elsewhere. He felt no compulsion to achieve prestige or win awards like his father. Like the man whose letter he held in his hand, he wanted to make great discoveries. Even after four years of severe discipline and bloody conflict, his mind wandered to the problem that consumed him. All of his earlier work—consisting of a body most would be proud to achieve in a lifetime—had been preparation for the problem he wanted to attach his name to forever: cancer. He wanted to be the man who *cured* cancer.

Maybe it was the fact that he knew the war was over. Germany had lost. Like so many decisive moments in history, it wasn't the force of the message alone but also the context it fell into. Whether from his ambitions, the letter, homesickness, or an amalgam of everything, he packed his bags. He looked at his Iron Cross First Class and thought about the wounds he had received in action. He may not get another chance. His uncle, a general on a different front, had been killed. When later asked about the war, Warburg said, "I was taught that one must be more than one appears to be."

After the war, unlike most of Europe's youth, Warburg had something remarkable to go home to. Just months before he volunteered for the army, he had been appointed a member of the Kaiser-Wilhelm-Gesellschaft zur Förderung der Wissenschaften (Kaiser Wilhelm Society for the Advancement of Science). The scientific institution independent of the state acquired funding from international sources including the American Rockefeller Institute. This was no ordinary appointment. The institute prescribed to a model where a few carefully selected scientists were made "members." The title was reserved for minds to be set free, deemed worthy of such an appointment. With member status came high pay, no distractions, and no teaching or administrative responsibilities. As Warburg's former teacher, Emil Fisher, described it, "You will be completely independent. No one will ever trouble you. No one will ever interfere. You may walk in the woods for a few years or, if you like, may ponder over something beautiful."

Today, the best American scientists spend over half their time applying for grants. The strategy paid enormous dividends for Germany and the world as a whole. With members like Albert Einstein, the scientists made massive scientific leaps forward. On the top floor of a building in the heart of Berlin, a laboratory was waiting.

Warburg was born October 8, 1883, in Freiburg, a picturesque town nestled on the western edge of Germany's vaunted Black Forest.

How Cancer Became Known as a Genetic Disease

The town was rife with Bavarian charm and a rich, intellectual history stemming from one of Germany's oldest universities. He was the only boy in the family, had three sisters, and exhibited a mischievous side as a school boy. A letter written to his parents when he was thirteen admonished his behavior for "inciting fellow pupils to take part in gross misconduct." When interviewed, he did what most boys would do: he lied. It was suggested in the letter that "these bad traits be energetically dealt with at home." It is doubtful that they were. His father, Emil Warburg, was distant, although successful in his academic career. According to Warburg's sisters, he had little interest in people.

It didn't matter that his parents didn't "energetically deal" with his untruthfulness at school. In time, he would come to covet truth and discipline as the most important qualities a person could possess. Maybe it was the dinner guests of his childhood home, a virtual who's who list of the "Grand Masters" of science in an era of remarkable achievement. Perhaps they combined to shape the personality of young Otto. Through his father, Warburg got to know Emil Fisher, the leading organic chemist of his day; Walter Nernst, the leading physical chemist; and others including Max Plank and Albert Einstein, who later became Warburg's close friend.

His ambitions became obvious early. He wanted to be a great scientist. In the time-honored question of nature versus nurture, both sides of the equation were tilted in Warburg's favor. He was reared by brilliant parents, imbued with a desire to discover, and shaped during his formative years by the best scientists in the world.

Warburg learned physics and chemistry from his father and his colleagues. He was taught chemistry from Nernst and learned physics in the laboratory of his father. At eighteen, he began his studies in chemistry at the University of Freiburg. As was customary in central Europe, he moved to another university at Berlin, where he completed his doctoral thesis under Fisher in 1906. His interests began to shift from the physical sciences toward medicine, he discovered that he had an intense curiosity about how the body worked – and didn't work. He was inspired to understand pathology, the branch of medicine focusing on how things went wrong. Always one to embrace challenges and never sidestep big issues, he was naturally drawn to the problem of cancer.

And so in a surprising shift from the stern physical science atmosphere in which he was reared, he enrolled in medical school at Heidelberg University. He thrived in the new atmosphere. The collision between his physical science background and his interest in pathology proved advantageous, because he was able to approach medicine from the unique angle of a physical scientist. The work ethic instilled in him by his father remained, when he wasn't studying, he filled his spare time working in the laboratory of the department of internal medicine. He graduated with his MD in the spring of 1911. A harbinger of his potential, he published no less than thirty important papers while working in his spare time during medical school and in the few years after his graduation. But as prodigious as his research had been, all of it was just a strategic prelude – a preparation for what was next – his effort to discover the nature of cancer.

While working in Heidelberg, he received notice that he had been granted member status to the Gesellschaft. The appointment would give him unprecedented resources to attack cancer with, but it would have to wait. Unfortunatly his innate desire to tackle big issues head on included the war that was about to break out. In 1914, three years after graduating from medical school, on the cusp of shifting his focus to cancer, he volunteered to go to war on behalf of his country. Almost a decade would pass before he again turned his attention to cancer.

Once the war was over and he settled into a new position at the institute, for the first time in his life Warburg was able to exclusively focus on cancer. As a biochemist, he spoke a different language from most. To him, cancer could be defined only in strict molecular terms, the words of the material universe. It could be described only by dissecting it to the atomic level – penetrating the heart of the disease. He felt that the most fundamental operation of the cell, or life in general, was the creation of energy. Life was a surreal oasis of order in a universe that tended toward disorder. From the moment of our birth our bodies were thrust into a losing battle; forced, without a moment's rest, to create energy just to keep the relentless force of entropy at bay. Energy alone keeps us whole, without it, we dissolved back into the elements from which we came. Growing, reproducing, moving, thinking, and communicating—everything depended on the continuous creation of energy. If the metabolic generation of energy was cut off, it was only a matter of minutes before the organism died.

Warburg's conviction that cancer was an energy problem was anchored in the nonspecific nature of the disease. Most diseases were specific. If you got infected by tuberculosis, it manifested as a respiratory disease. If your circulatory system became clogged, it manifested as a heart attack or a stroke. Warburg felt that cancer was more fundamental. It had countless causes, as Pott and Rous had discovered, and it could erupt from any tissue, as any physician could attest to. It was a fundamental problem, and nothing was more fundamental to life than energy.

At the time, it was known that human cells used oxygen to create energy. The French scientist Louis Pasteur, whom Warburg admired, termed this type of energy creation *aerobic* (also called respiration). The other type was without oxygen and with the formation of lactic acid, and Pasteur termed this *anaerobic*. Anaerobic energy creation (also called fermentation) was a primordial pathway that extracted a fraction of the intrinsic energy within a molecule of glucose. Because life flickered into existence in an atmosphere with no oxygen, fermentation was the first pathway to evolve. It is conserved across a broad span of living things from humans to monkeys, birds, yeast, spinach, bacteria, and everything between. But the pathway is extremely inefficient. It takes eighteen times more glucose to extract the same amount of energy from fermentation than from respiration. If the two pathways, aerobic and anaerobic, were represented by cars, the only difference being the motor, the aerobic model would get 38 miles per gallon, and the anaerobic model would get 2 miles per gallon.

As organisms climbed the evolutionary ladder toward complexity and specialization, aerobic energy metabolism took over. A normal human cell typically obtains almost 90 percent of its energy by aerobic metabolism and the remainder through an anaerobic pathway. It was also known at the time that cells were hardwired with an adaptive mechanism. Certain cells, like muscle cells, could create energy without oxygen, generating lactic acid but only briefly when oxygen was absent or the muscles demanded great amounts of energy. Once oxygen was added or the activity stopped, the cells resumed the much more efficient method of making energy aerobically.

In 1908, while still in medical school, Warburg began making observations about the energetic requirements of dividing sea urchin eggs. He found that the large eggs were a good model to study because they were easy to work with and fertilization sparked a furious eruption of cell division, reflecting the type of hyper growth seen in malignancy. He reasoned that the explosion of cell division must be driven by a commensurate increase in energy creation. His measurements proved his logic was sound. The rate of oxygen consumption within the sea urchin eggs increased six fold upon fertilization. The eggs underwent a massive burst of respiration to fuel the rapid growth.

The sea urchin model of cell proliferation was in the back of Warburg's mind when he began to investigate cancer. He guessed cancer probably mirrored the explosive growth of the sea urchin embryo, and therefore, like the sea urchin embryo, must also greatly increase the consumption of oxygen in order to supply the energy necessary for such growth. He pioneered vastly improved techniques with which to approach the question, and his results were the highest quality. He used thin slices of tissue in culture, which allowed him to perform experiments with intact cells in their normal matrix of surrounding tissue. He drew upon his background in physics to adapt a state-of-the-art manometer and measure the rate of gas exchange. This was critical to quantifying the delicate difference of oxygen exchange between cancer cells and normal cells.

When Warburg began his investigation he noticed something striking. Even though cancer cells exhibited the same kind of explosive growth as the sea urchin eggs, they didn't fuel it through increased respiration alone. To Warburg's surprise, cancer cells generated abnormal amounts of lactic acid. They were generating energy through the antiquated fermentation pathway, and even more surprising, they did it in the presence of oxygen. True to his meticulous nature, he set out to ensure that the observation was unique to cancer cells. He tested different tissues to see if any could ferment in the presence of oxygen, but none of them did. This led to Warburg's famous distinction: unlike normal cells, cancer cells fermented glucose in the presence of oxygen, a quality now simply known as "the Warburg effect."

He also noted that cancer cells did not produce more or less energy than normal cells; they just produced it in a different way. For example, a cancer cell might produce 40 percent of its energy aerobically and 60 percent anaerobically, but the total added up to the same amount as a normal cell. Cancer cells were producing energy in a way that evolution had set aside as an auxiliary pathway, a highly inefficient generator that kicked in when the power went out.

As Warburg continued his experiments with various types of tumor cells, he found that cancer's defective metabolism presented itself without exception. Now he could be sure. To him, this was the prime cause into which all other secondary causes collapsed. The reversion from aerobic to anaerobic energy generation was the signature that defined the difference between cancer cells and normal cells. Nothing was more fundamental to a cell than energy creation. Nothing could be further reduced.

Years later, Warburg made another critical observation that hinted at why cancer cells were fermenting in the first place. He showed that when normal, healthy cells were deprived of oxygen for brief periods (hours) of time, they turned cancerous. No other carcinogens, viruses, or radiation were needed, just a lack of oxygen. This led him to conclude that cancer must be caused by "injury" to the cell's ability to respire. He contended that once damaged by lack of oxygen, the cell's respiratory machinery (later found to be mitochondria) became permanently broken and could not be rescued by returning the cells to an oxygen-rich environment. He reasoned that cancer must be caused by a permanent alteration to the respiratory machinery of the cell. It was a simple and elegant hypothesis. Warburg would contend until his death that this was the prime cause of cancer.

Pott's carcinogens, Rous's sarcoma virus, Hansemann's chaotic chromosomes, and Warburg's metabolic theory defined the understanding of cancer during the first half of the twentieth century. The competing theories jousted, coalesced, repelled each other, and fell in and out of favor as new evidence presented itself.

Hansemann's chaotic chromosomes by themselves were weakly correlative at best and did not definitively establish whether cause existed before or after effect. Did the broken chromosomes cause cancer, or were they merely a side effect? Hansemann certainly believed that they were the cause, but others needed more evidence. His idea that damaged chromosomes were the intrinsic force behind malignant growth became more powerful when it was combined with Pott's observation that external agents could cause cancer. The observations made a seductive pair, each buttressing the other and together forming the SMT of cancer.

As the twentieth century progressed, the idea that cancer originated from damage to chromosomes gained momentum. The idea that malicious agents were finding their way into the cells and rewiring genetic material had an intrinsic appeal to researchers. The combination was a siren call leading cancer researches to an intellectually satiating conclusion. The list of carcinogens only grew larger as time passed (today the list is 240 and counting). The only problem was that the theory had two unconnected dots. One was the observation that corrosive agents could cause cancer over time, and the other was how the agents were mutating or changing the chromosomal architecture in a way that precipitated the disease. Chromosomes were the prime suspect, but it was unclear how they were being damaged, and more importantly, how the damage resulted in uncontrolled growth. Without the techniques and instrumentation to determine the nature of chromosomal damage, the question remained unanswered. Until a direct line from carcinogen to alteration to uncontrolled proliferation could be drawn, the SMT was incomplete.

The context in which Rous discovered his cancer-causing chicken virus helped to anchor his fledgling viral theory into the minds of researchers and the public. In the decades that followed, the viral theory was present, but it faced the glaring fact that cancer-causing viruses had yet to be discovered in humans. They would have to be found at the scene of the crime, and an explanation was needed for how microscopic, otherworldly forms of parasitic life hijacked cellular machinery in a way that caused uncontrolled growth. Enough viruses had been discovered in other animals to keep the theory afloat. Rous's viral theory experienced many bouts of enthusiasm followed by disappointment, but it never went away.

Warburg's metabolic theory was the first to noticeably fade. In the beginning of the twentieth century, it was mentioned in journals as a curious aspect of cancer cells but nothing more. Although he continued to insist that damage to aerobic respiration was the origin of cancer, he was unable to convince others. And as the force of his reputation faded, so did his theory. As the SMT gained a stronger foothold Warburg's theory was further marginalized. His theory was questioned as early as 1928. G. Lenthal Cheatle, lecturer and surgeon at King's College Hospital in London wrote, "Even if Warburg is completely right [about the defective metabolism of the cancer cell], it does not explain why cancer cells grow." And that remained the main criticism of Warburg's theory. Injury to cellular respiration, as far as other researchers were concerned, was not linked to uncontrolled growth. In the minds of most, injury to chromosomes, the hereditary structures that dictated so many cellular functions, seemed the obvious culprit.

Without a comprehensive theory, the science on the origin of cancer was held captive between the competing theories, suspended in a theoretical standoff. But for the rest of cellular biology, the second half of the twentieth century was a time of incandescent discovery. As the century hit middle age, molecular biology came to dominate the headlines. A new generation of clever, young molecular biologists, armed with exciting new instruments and techniques, began defining life in new terms – sparking an explosive understanding of how cells operate.

Glimpse by glimpse, pixel by pixel, researchers pieced together an internal image of the cell, revealing all the functionality of a self-sufficient city. Diagrams depicting cellular function decorated the pages of biological journals like modern hieroglyphics of a bold, new era of self-discovery. The architecture of the cell was remarkably similar to a city. Food was imported, stored, and selectively metered out to power plants called mitochondria. A variety of fuels were combusted with oxygen inside the oval furnaces, churning out a common energetic currency that other workers throughout the cell could spend. Waste was sorted, packaged, dissolved, and exported. Researchers found out that cells were microeconomies with division and specialization of labor. They had elaborate communication systems that facilitated the flow of important information allowing the cell to adapt to changing environments.

The new image of the cell was one of a beautifully efficient, adaptable, and resourceful marvel of organization. A cell didn't exist in isolation but, like a city, was a hub of interdependent, bustling activity. The prosaic and dreary biology textbooks of the past were transformed into engaging books with colorful images of macromolecular symmetry exploding from the pages – visual feasts of the exquisite structure and form of life.

The Secret of Life

The seminal moment in the understanding of life came in the middle of the century. The cell was found to have a central "government" responsible for dictating and directing the operational landscape. Molecular biology's defining moment when a scientific field moved from darkness into illumination was about to occur. It began in Cambridge, England, when two tall, skinny, awkward-looking scientists were having a beer in a pub.

It was the winter of 1953. It was an overcast February day in England, the same as the day before and the day before that. The researchers in the Cavendish lab at Kings College knew how to deal with the dreary weather. Six days a week, they headed off to the Eagle Pub and shared lunch and an occasional pint. But today was different, because their years of effort had just paid off.

The American, James Watson, and the Englishman, Francis Crick, were in a fierce race with American scientist Linus Pauling to discover the structure of DNA, the molecule they suspected to be the blueprint of life. To determine its structure, the duo built model after model, arranging the molecules they knew it contained into various patterns. They finally built one that made sense and was in harmony with the laws of chemistry and physics. As they stared at it from every angle, Watson said, "It was too beautiful to not be it." But still a small part of him had reservations. He wanted to be absolutely sure, so he held back his excitement for one more test to put the final stamp of approval on it. However the outspoken and fiercely confident Englishman, Crick, needed nothing more. He knew they had nailed it. He felt it in his gut.

When Crick walked into the Eagle to find his colleagues sitting against the far wall, pints half drained, he couldn't contain his enthusiasm any longer. "We discovered the secret of life!" he announced to every patron within earshot.

It was beautiful. It was two strands of sugar and phosphate twirling around each other, forming a perfect double helix—a striking portrait of nature's bend toward symmetry. In the middle of the strands was a series of four molecules that bound in an exact pattern, zipping the strands together. Far more important than the pleasing form of the molecule were the implications embedded in the structure. There is a saying that held true across the spectrum of biology: structure equaled function. Crick said it this way: "If you want to understand function, study structure." It is true for your eyes, your thumb, and your big toe. Every part of your body was sculpted through a crucible of trial and error, and it was no different for DNA. The code for life was hidden inside the beautiful molecule. Everything from self-awareness to the color of hair on your head is written in the double helix.

The years to come revealed how the information within DNA was translated into action. The *New York Times* labeled the years from 1953 to 1966 the "golden age of molecular biology when the high mysteries of the genetic code and protein synthesis were worked out." Scientists revealed the code hidden within the molecules that zipped up the double helix: adenine, guanine, thymine, and cytosine. They were called base pairs, because without exception, they interacted in pairs—guanine with cytosine and adenine with thymine. It wasn't the base pairs themselves that were significant; it was their order. They acted no differently than the binary code a computer used. By themselves they were meaningless, but collectively, lined up within the swirling helix, they contained all the information of life. In his book *What Is Life?* the great physicist Erwin Schrodinger concluded, "The essence of life is information." Now scientists knew where the information was stored.

The intricate operations of the cell are carried out by legions of workers called proteins. They are the workhorses. Proteins provide the supportive scaffolding of the cell. Proteins even dictate the structure of DNA itself, tightly winding it in a superstructure of coils wrapped within coils. In some sections, DNA directs the proteins to "stay away," allowing designated sections of DNA (genes) to be exposed. Other sections are tightly hidden away, allowing each cell type to express a defined set of genes – a phenomenon known as cell specialization. Directed by a continuous dance between DNA and the environment, proteins dictate the three-dimensional architecture of DNA, allowing for specialization and adaption. In a hair follicle, for example, the gene encoding for the hair protein is exposed, but in a liver cell, it is wrapped up. Proteins act as gateways, directing materials into and out of the cell. They serve as catalysts, facilitating myriad chemical reactions that continuously generate energy and power an almost inconceivable number of cellular processes. Proteins function as intricate circuit boards within the cell. They constantly receive signals from the outside in the form of hormones or nutrients, and then relay the information through the appropriate channels, always adjusting and adapting. The cell is a dynamic symphony of activity, all facilitated through the action of proteins.

Proteins are originally manufactured as a linear string. A strand is comprised of a series of smaller subunit molecules called amino acids (twenty-one of them). Like words in a sentence, it is the order that matters. The order of the amino acids determines the ultimate function of the protein. The order of amino acids dictates whether the protein ends up being a receptor for insulin positioned on the outside of the cellular membrane or to be insulin itself. The placement of amino acids determines how the linear string of amino acids folds in on itself in the aqueous solution of the cell. Certain amino acids don't dissolve well in water, like oil droplets suspended on the surface of a pond. Oil-like amino acids fold into the middle of the protein, trying to escape the water surrounding them. They are called hydrophobic amino acids precisely because of their phobia of water. The amino acids that do dissolve well in water (*hydrophilic* or "water loving") are left on the surface. Again, structure equals function, so the three-dimensional architecture of the protein—once it collapses in on itself, conforming to its most "comfortable" position—determines its job. Just as a lawnmower and a car are made from the same materials (metal, plastic, rubber, and so on), every protein is made of the same twenty-one amino acids, but the different configurations allow them to serve vastly different functions.

Coming back to DNA, the pattern, or code of the base pairs of DNA, determines the order of the amino acids in a given protein. A unit of three base pairs, called a codon, calls for one of the twenty-one amino acids. Large, industrial-like proteins travel along DNA, reading each codon as they go and translating the information into a messenger molecule called messenger RNA (mRNA). The mRNA serves as an intermediary between DNA and proteins, like a pigeon carrying a letter. Another large protein then attaches to mRNA, reading it codon by codon, picking out the amino acids designated by each codon, and stitching them together to form a protein. This is the code of life. The flow of information in biological systems is a one-way street from DNA to RNA to protein. Crick called the process "the central dogma of biology." The DNA code for a section of insulin looks like this: C C A T A G C A C G T T A C A A C G T G A A G G T A A.

After Watson and Crick revealed the molecule at the center of the biological universe, all lights pointed at DNA. Researchers were captivated by its elegance and power. DNA was life, and the rest of us—from amoebas and blowfish to higher primates and man—were just pawns doing its bidding. It was calling the shots. We were nothing more than temporal experiments. We were experimental shells designed to see how well a given code performed within a given environment. Distilled to its essence, and all philosophical or religious precepts set aside, life is code. The codes that prove well suited to the environment they inhabit tend to reproduce. Other codes fall by the wayside as failed experiments. From its lowly prebiotic origin some four billion years ago, DNA adapted and morphed into an explosion of life, filling every niche on the planet from the boiling pools in Yellowstone National Park to the Arctic shelf. Life is everywhere.

It wasn't surprising that cancer researchers soon became spellbound by DNA as well. If the code of DNA dictated *all* the functionality of an organism, alterations within the code probably caused cellular behavior to go awry. To imagine that alterations to DNA could manifest in cancer was easy. Now the connection between Hansemann's broken chromosomes and Pott's carcinogens seemed obvious. By the 1960s, the idea that DNA was central to cancer was widely accepted.

Frank Horsfall, MD, vice president and physician in chief of the Rockefeller Institute, gave a presentation in the fall of 1963 titled "Current Concepts of Cancer." It was part of a commencement celebrating fifty years of medical education at one of Canada's premier medical schools (the University of Alberta), and the speech summarized the thoughts regarding the origin of cancer at the time and the central role of DNA. "Because the cancerous change in cells appears to be a permanent alteration, handed on to daughter cells through innumerable divisions, it seems probable that it reflects an abnormality in the transfer of information from cell to daughter cells. Transfer of information in cells is believed to depend on their genetic apparatus, and transfer of abnormal information implies that the genetic apparatus is not functioning normally."

All the evidence pointed to alterations in DNA as the origin of the disease, but researchers had yet to see the alterations. They still didn't know how DNA was being altered or which genes were altered. They had a pile of circumstantial evidence to suggest that it *was* being altered, but the details remained elusive. The pesky viral theory, championed by Rous, was still a misshapen puzzle piece that prevented a grand unification of all observation into a comprehensive theory. It was known that viruses inserted chunks of DNA into the genomes of infected cells, but it was not known what these chunks looked like or how they acted. Were they some sort of foreign viral code that transformed a normal cell into a cancerous one? Was it encoding for a protein, or numerous proteins, that could subvert the steady-state operations of the cell into uncontrolled proliferators? Where did the viruses get their transforming chunks of DNA? How widespread were these viral chunks of DNA? Did everybody carry them unknowingly? Were they passed through the germline from parent to offspring? If they were already there, did other carcinogens serve as agents that activated viral DNA?

Researchers felt that DNA was involved in the origin of cancer, but in what manner? In the years leading up to the 1960s, virologists had finally found a virus suspected of causing cancer in man, but many questions remained.

But all that was about to change. Any lingering questions about the origin of cancer were about to be answered by a remarkable series of experiments that defined cancer as we know it today.

A Question That Had Passed Him By

On a summer day in 1966, at age eighty-two, Warburg took the podium to give what would be his final address and summary of his life's research on cancer. The title of his lecture was "On the Primary Causes and on the Secondary Causes of Cancer." When he took the podium, he knew that he was in an awkward situation. He realized he very well may have been the last scientist to believe that cancer was metabolic in nature, precipitating from irreversible damage to the mitochondria (the oval structures that floated throughout the cell's interior discovered to be responsible for generating energy through respiration twenty years earlier).

He was speaking to a distinguished crowd. The occasion was the annual gathering of Nobel laureates at Lindau, Germany, a red-roofed medieval town nestled on an island on the eastern shore of Lake Constance. The gathering began as a post-World War II effort to rouse German doctors and scientists out of hiding, giving them a peaceful reason to return to Germany and begin anew. The beacon worked, and from the corners of the globe, they came back to rekindle the vibrant intellectual culture that permeated prewar Germany. Warburg, among a handful of others, perhaps epitomized the rich scientific culture that Germany nurtured before the war—a "golden age" of science. A mutual friend of the Lindau meeting's founders used his contacts with the Swedish royal family and the Nobel committee in Stockholm, persuading them to help expand the original vision into something more—an annual gathering of all the World's Nobel Laureates, side by side, with the next generation of young scientists, a meeting that arched across generations, nationalities, and scientific disciplines.

Warburg cleared his throat, scanned the audience with his piercing, blue eyes, and began to speak. His delivery retained the force and clarity he was known for. Even among a crowd of Nobel laureates, he stood out. His career had been remarkably productive. He won a Nobel Prize in 1931 for work describing how cells used oxygen to create energy. He was nominated for the Nobel Prize three separate times for three separate achievements. None of the laureates in the crowd could equal this. Indeed most in the audience considered him the greatest biochemist of the twentieth century (as did Warburg himself). He had acquired a reputation for his unwavering conviction and belief in his assertions, a trait often perceived as arrogance. Many felt that he was unreasonably stubborn and picked fights without provocation. Certainly he did not suffer fools gladly. He felt that as a biochemist, he towered above everyone else, and he felt that he alone carried on where the great Pasteur left off (Pasteur was also a chemist turned biologist). When it was announced that he won the Nobel Prize in 1931, his reaction was, "It's high time."

Even if some had conflicting feelings about his personality, he inspired an emotion that infected the audience: respect. Even those who didn't like him had to respect him. He had single-handedly thrust the understanding of cellular physiology ahead by leaps and bounds. Even though the breadth of his achievement was vast, one question cut through the center of it: what was the origin of cancer? Ironically, the question that he wanted to answer the most was the one that others in the audience felt had passed him by. To them, it was the asterisk on his remarkable career. But true to his nature, he didn't back down. In his mind, he had answered the question, and everyone else could be damned. He knew in his gut that he was right and would be vindicated in the end.

He was sure that he had found the prime cause of cancer more than forty years earlier: the cellular event to which all secondary causes converged. His speech could be distilled into three succinct sentences: "Cancer, above all other diseases, has countless secondary causes. Almost anything can cause cancer, but even for cancer, there is only one prime cause. The prime cause of cancer is the replacement of the respiration of oxygen in normal body cells by fermentation of sugar."

This single perversion of energy generation, Warburg staunchly believed, was the cause of cancer. Secondary causes such as x-rays, dyes, tar, asbestos, and cigarette smoke were largely irrelevant. They only precipitated the prime cause: damaged respiration.

Other biologists in the audience were convinced that Warburg's hypothesis was wrong and that it was barely propped up by an old man who was unable to keep up with his own fast-moving discipline. Every scientist eventually gets to this point—sloughed off like a dead layer of skin as a new generation pushed up from the bottom. They listened politely. Even though they felt he was wrong, he had banked their goodwill and respect. He had earned the podium.

That night, Warburg sat in a chair in a hotel room. The Lindau meeting was over, and it was late, but he couldn't sleep. Like most old men, he let his mind wander too far into the past. He knew that his colleagues had designated him a dinosaur—he could tell by their expressions, the response to his speech, and the conversations afterward. He knew that he was right about the origin of cancer, an instinct honed from a lifetime of discovery, but he was tired of trying to convince them. They would find out on their own. He rose from his chair, turned out the light, and went to sleep.

On July 24, 1970, Warburg didn't feel well. The next day, he felt a sharp pain in his leg where he had sustained a fracture two years prior falling off the ladder in his library while putting away a book. He stayed home the rest of the week, reading and writing. On August 1, he woke up feeling weak. Later that evening, at age eighty-seven, he died. He had never married or had children. His work was the only thing that survived him. Everybody thought that, unlike the majority of his work, his theory on the origin of cancer had died with him.

Everything Was in a Fog

Harold Varmus didn't set off to become a research scientist. Far from it. To get there, he wandered a circuitous path. When he enrolled at Amherst College in 1957, he intended to become a medical doctor like his father, but the sixties were right around the corner, and he soon found himself way off the premed track. "I was more enamored with Keynesian novels, metaphysical poetry, and anti-establishment journalism than my premedical studies." So he changed his major to English literature and received his BA in 1961. At Harvard, he earned a graduate degree in English in 1962, but halfway through his first year, a dream sent him back full circle. As he described in a 2006 interview with Richard Poynder, he dreamed that he had become an English professor and that he had to miss a day of lecture due to illness. Instead of being disappointed, his students were ecstatic that class was canceled. When he woke, he realized that if he became a physician, no one would be happy if he didn't show up for work. The epiphany sent him back to where he began, and he applied to medical school. After getting rejected from Harvard twice, he landed at Columbia University and earned his medical degree. He had to decide what kind of doctor he wanted to be, and his capricious nature again reared its head. "I had an interest, I hate to admit it, in psychiatry," he later said. After coming to his senses, he chose internal medicine. Later he realized that his convoluted career path came close to impeding a meaningful career in science, admitting that he became committed to experimental science "dangerously late in a prolonged adolescence." But his commitment to science came all at once when, as an intern, he picked up the *Journal of Molecular Biology* at Columbia-Presbyterian Hospital and began reading. "I knew from that moment, my life had changed," he later said in his Nobel Prize acceptance speech. He was hooked.

The timing was perfect. In 1968, rather than serving in the Vietnam War, he signed up for the public health service at NIH. It was the perfect home for an MD suddenly fascinated by molecular biology. He was able to learn the technical craft of molecular biology, and when the laboratory work was finished for the day, he attended evening classes designed to expose researchers to exciting new fields and ideas. One class focused on the exploding field of tumor viruses, and it captivated his imagination. It planted a seed that incubated in his subconscious. A detective might call it a hunch, but he felt that the answer to cancer lay in the tiniest of life forms: cancer-causing viruses.

Whatever gut instinct led Varmus to tumor viruses, it was also a stroke of good fortune, because to any researcher interested in the genetics of cancer, viruses, as Varmus confessed, "were really the only game in town." With the rudimentary technology in the 1970s, tumor viruses, with their simple genomes and capacity to be manipulated experimentally, were the best hope for a biologist trying to learn about the genetics of cancer.

Varmus set out to look where he could, but first he needed a lab, a suitable place to study tumor viruses. Colleagues tipped him off to a small group working with the Rous sarcoma virus (RSV) in San Francisco. In the summer of 1969, Varmus and a colleague combined a backpacking trip with his plan to drop in on the San Francisco group and size up the laboratory as a potential home. The scientist Varmus was supposed to meet wasn't there, and he met Michael Bishop instead. "A brief conversation with Mike was sufficient to convince me of our intellectual compatibility," said Varmus. The connection between

Varmus and Bishop was instant and powerful. Both were free spirited and both were intensely interested in how viruses caused cancer. Varmus knew he was home, and he made plans to join the group as a postdoctoral fellow the following summer. In a 2006 interview with *Wired,* Varmus described the working relationship that developed with Bishop over the years. "The research I did with Mike didn't have the manic quality of some scientific discoveries, like the discovery of the double helix. This was Wagner rather than Mozart—a slow elaboration of themes, sung over and over again."

Their goal to understand the transforming power of tumor viruses was first in the order of importance to establish an all-encompassing genetic theory of cancer. As Horsfall suggested in his speech more than a decade before, researchers knew that DNA was involved in cancer, but tumor viruses were the unknown. They didn't fit anywhere— nobody knew how they worked, how prevalent they were, or how they ultimately caused cancer. Researchers proposed two theories describing how viruses might be causing cancer. The first, called the viral gene oncogene hypothesis, proposed that we all carry ancient viral genes in our germline DNA, passing it on from parent to offspring. These foreign genes could then be activated by carcinogens, thus precipitating cancer. The second theory was called the provirus hypothesis. It contended that viral genes were not permanently integrated into our DNA, passed down over generations, but were inserted upon viral infection, only then precipitating cancer. Varmus and Bishop set out to discover which theory was correct.

First they needed to isolate which one of the RSV genes was responsible for turning a normal cell cancerous. It was not a trivial task but was made easier by the simplicity of RSV, which contained only four genes. In a stroke of good fortune, another lab did the work for them, isolating the transforming ability of RSV down to a single gene. They named the cancer-causing gene src (for sarcoma).

They were able to skip ahead to the task of determining how this single viral gene was causing cancer. To do this they would have to understand the nature of the gene. Was it an exotic viral gene with no resemblance to anything in the animal kingdom, or did it rhyme with one of our own genes? It would be an exercise in comparison. By itself the code of the viral gene was meaningless, but if it could be compared to other genes for which the function was known, they might gain some insight into how the src gene was acting. The symmetrical structure of DNA itself provided the solution. Because the code of DNA consisted of base pairs that always bonded in the same pattern (C with T and A with G), a single strand of DNA could be used as a sort of molecular fishing pole.

Varmus and Bishop used a special protein to copy the genetic code of the viral genome to use as bait: a single strand of DNA. They erased the three genes of RSV not responsible for cancer, leaving the src gene behind. Because it was single stranded, the nucleotides no longer existed as pairs. They were left hanging, suspended in space, yearning to bind to their counterparts like a single piece of Velcro looking for its partner. The single-stranded bait was radio labeled so that it could be "seen" once it "caught" its counterpart. All that was left was to go fishing. The idea was simple: if anything resembling the src gene was found in the genome of other animals, they would gain insight into the nature of src.

They started their molecular "fishing trip" in other species of birds. To their surprise, their fishing pole caught its genetic counterpart in every bird they tested—the viral src gene was more widespread than they had imagined. They experienced instant and powerful bites, as the nucleotides left as bait found their virtual exact counterpart. They moved on to other species. To their amazement, everywhere they fished, they caught the src gene: in fish, rabbits, mice, cows, sheep, and humans. The cancer-causing gene in RSV was an essential gene to life. It was not some arcane and mysterious viral gene. Src was already part of us.

The research duo had to rule out the possibility that they were simply detecting the RSV itself traveling across species lines. Maybe the chicken virus was wildly infectious. To eliminate this possibility, they designed another radio-labeled probe with the rest of the Rous viral genome, the other three genes they had erased earlier in order to isolate the src gene. This time when they went fishing in other birds, they didn't find anything. Nor did they find anything in the other species tested, including humans.

This confirmed that RSV was not a viral pandemic that spanned the animal kingdom, and the implications were profound. The cancer-causing gene of RSV was a distorted copy of a common gene that is in all species, part of our inherited DNA, not caused by some foreign piece of DNA inserted into us by the virus. When Varmus gave his Noble Prize lecture in 1989, he said, "I soon learned how much more important a new measurement was than an old theory." The implication of this new measurement would change everything. Viral DNA was not embedded in all of us, waiting for activation by carcinogens, as some had suggested. The cancer-causing portion of viral DNA was a distorted version of the DNA we already had.

The gene that was responsible for the cancer-causing ability in the virus discovered by Rous nearly seventy years before was in all of us. The "fishing pole" they constructed was able to detect the normal version of the src gene, because the viral, cancer-causing version was only subtly different from the normal version. The majority of the hanging nucleotides on the src fishing pole matched up with the cellular version allowing it to be detected. The few nucleotides that did not match up were responsible for turning the normal version of the gene (proto-oncogene) into a cancer-causing version (oncogene). It had been known for some time that viruses were genetic thieves, pirating genes of the host they infected and incorporating the code into their own genome. RSV was no different—it had stolen the src gene.

Researchers began looking at the few nucleotides that were altered in the viral version of the src gene. The alterations exposed how the normal gene was malevolently corrupted. The protein biochemists took over. They discovered the normal version of src encoded for a protein known as a kinase.

Kinases typically fall into the category of signaling molecules—they are the chatty version of proteins, continuously relaying information throughout the cell. They transfer signals by adding a phosphate group onto a designated protein, slightly altering its three-dimensional architecture and thus its function. Cellular communication is a tightly regulated process that required kinases to have "on" and "off" switches. The protein biochemists found that the viral version of src was a kinase with its brake line cut. The mutations in the nucleotide code of the viral version, in the end, slightly altered the amino acid sequence of the protein, a sequence change that substantially altered its function. The protein product of the viral src version was stuck in the "on" position—it attached phosphates to other proteins with reckless abandon like a person yelling "Fire!" in a packed movie theater. The normal cellular version remained in control; it could be turned off. Because the viral version was stuck in the "on" position, it continuously shouted the instructions for the cell to divide over and over again.

The discovery was an epiphany. Cancer researchers finally knew that viruses caused cancer by capturing a normal cellular gene, slightly altering it, and inserting the slightly distorted version of our own gene into our DNA. Another possibility was that the cancer-causing virus didn't even have to alter the normal src gene while in its custody. The virus may have stolen the distorted src gene from a cancer cell itself. One of Pott's carcinogens, or some other mutational process, may have altered the src gene of some poor unknowing chicken. RSV happened to then steal and incorporate the cancer-causing version directly into its DNA. What was a normal, probably inconsequential virus was now a tumor virus. Loaded with the new oncogene, the virus unknowingly redistributed the oncogene upon infection—a cancerous version of Typhoid Mary.

Src was a signaling molecule that was out of control. Now there was no question about how Pott's carcinogens acted. They acted like the virus, altering the genes responsible for cellular proliferation by turning proto-oncogenes into oncogenes. Proto-oncogenes were normal genes responsible for controlling cellular growth, but because of Varmus and Bishop's experiment, they now represented vulnerability. Now proto-oncogenes appeared like land mines, sprinkled throughout our genomes, waiting to be set off. Proto-oncogenes were seeds baked into our bodies, lying dormant until germinated from a carcinogen or reinserted by a tumor virus.

Hansemann's chaotic chromosomes were simply a visual manifestation of the process whether the cause was through carcinogens or a virus. In an instant, Rous's pesky viral theory of cancer was unceremoniously recruited into the SMT. Varmus and Bishop's discovery stitched the patchwork of evidence into a unified whole. A number of disparate observations were connected. As acclaimed author and cancer researcher Siddhartha Mukherjee put it, "It was like watching a puzzle solve itself." Watson and Crick revealed the molecule at the center of the biological universe, and Varmus and Bishop showed that cancer was caused by alterations to it, leading to defective protein products. These protein products sabotaged the tight controls of orderly cell division, unleashing chaotic, uncontrolled proliferation. "It is not easy to convey, unless one has experienced it, the dramatic feeling of sudden enlightenment that floods the mind when the right idea finally clicks into place. One immediately sees how many previously puzzling facts are neatly explained by the new hypothesis. One could kick oneself for not having the idea earlier, it now seems so obvious. Yet before, everything was in a fog," Crick wrote.

After centuries of struggle, generations of effort, and too many casualties to count, mankind had the answer to one of its oldest and most relentless mysteries: the cause of cancer. The SMT of cancer was cast in iron. With Warburg dead and Rous's virus almost conspiratorially subverted into evidence for the SMT, no one was left to dispute it. The door slammed shut, and few would look back.

Part 2

Chemotherapy and the Gates of Hell

Embedded in the struggle to treat cancer was a narrative of our efforts to know cancer—to understand its paradoxical personality, to learn its strengths, neurosis, addictions, patterns, methods of operation, and weaknesses. Even though the science of cancer biology and therapeutic intervention were separate topics, they were also tangled together. The path had not always been linear with therapies following basic science. Sometimes the path was reversed when a basic understanding of cancer was revealed by therapeutic intervention.

The first attempts to treat cancer with drugs came from a time when researchers knew little of cancer's nature. The story of how these drugs came into existence was both shocking and instructive. Without question, these indiscriminate poisons, still largely in use today, shaped our perception of the disease. The story began in an unsuspecting place as far removed from a laboratory as one could imagine. Fittingly, and maybe ironically, chemotherapy was born out of a horrific scene that unfolded one night in the mists of World War II.

On December 3, 1943, Lieutenant Colonel Stewart Francis Alexander received a call and was told to pack his bags as quickly as possible. A plane was waiting for him. He was given a concise briefing. Three days before, the Germans had bombed the port of Bari in southern Italy, an important hub for the Allied forces. The Allies were caught by surprise; it was thought that the Luftwaffe was stretched too thin to pull off such an attack, and as a consequence, nobody was prepared. The lights were even left on for the Germans.

As the bombs began to fall from the sky, a horrific scene unfolded. The initial attack killed a thousand Allied servicemen. Hundreds of sailors jumped into the water to escape the sinking ships, and when they emerged, covered in an oily amalgam from the destroyed and leaking ships, many noticed a garlic-like odor. Strange symptoms begin to afflict them. Many complained of a burning sensation but didn't make the association between the oily mixture saturating their uniforms and clinging to their skin, perhaps thinking it was engine oil. As late afternoon turned into evening, they continued to complain that their skin was burning. The medical staff noticed that blisters began to form. Worse symptoms developed throughout the night. In addition to the burning skin, hundreds of soldiers went blind. The Allied high command knew what was causing the symptoms. That was why they called Alexander, but they had received orders from the top to keep it quiet.

Alexander arrived the next day. As he examined the patients and listened to the detailed accounts, he recognized the symptoms: burning skin, blindness, garlic-like odor. It had to be mustard gas. He was part of a team trained in the effects of war gases. Without delay, he told the medical staff how to treat the suffering soldiers, but when he approached the chain of command with his assessment, he was greeted with a wall of silence. He was told to carry on with his job, treat the men, and keep silent about what he knew. It was clear to him that the Allies were trying to cover up the fact that it was one of their own ships that was packed full of mustard gas. In the weeks that followed, eighty-three soldiers died from the toxic "friendly fire." The civilian deaths from the airborne cloud of gas that smoldered over the nearby towns went untallied, although many estimated it to be as many as one thousand.

Much later, it would be revealed that of the twenty-eight destroyed ships, the SS *John Harvey* was responsible. The entirety of its contents was released by the German bombs. More than 120,000 pounds of the yellow gas spilled into the bay or wafted into the ocean breeze, indiscriminately cast upon unsuspecting civilians. The Allied command covered it up because of the tenuous agreement by both sides to not use war gases. But neither side trusted the other, both were stockpiling mustard gas and prepared to retaliate.

It was impossible to accurately determine how many lives Alexander saved, or to quantify the degree of suffering he relieved by his intervention. He would receive recognition for this later, once the veil of secrecy surrounding the accident lifted. But it was what he carried in his bags when he returned home that he would be remembered for. His bags were packed full of tissue samples from the fallen victims.

Once home, doctors got to work analyzing the samples. One consistent feature stood out. The samples displayed a striking depletion of white blood cells within the lymph nodes and bone marrow, precisely the tissues that become packed with the feverishly dividing cells of lymphoma patients. Two Yale doctors, Louis Goodman and Alfred Gilman, who had contracted to study the therapeutic effects of nitrogen mustard, made the connection. In a short leap of imagination they entertained the possibility that the war gas possessed a strange dual nature, a Jekyll-and-Hyde compound that could exist both on the battlefield and within a physician's clinic. It was a long shot, but they convinced themselves that it was worth a try. They plotted a bizarre course to test the bizarre idea that the war gas might be a long-imagined chemotherapeutic agent.

They started with mice, and a series of experiments confirmed their hypothesis: it was clear that the mustard compound significantly regressed lymphoid tumors in mice. What started as a sliver of a possibility now seemed much less crazy. They were infected with the exciting realization they might have discovered a drug to fight cancer.

The pharmacologists then approached Gustaf Lindskog, a thoracic surgeon, asking him to help them with the next step. As crazy as it sounded, they asked him to administer nitrogen mustard to a lymphoma patient. After showing him the impressive preclinical mouse data, he finally agreed. The first patient Lindskog injected had non-Hodgkin's lymphoma accompanied with severe airway obstruction. It was an advanced case, and all options were exhausted. To their amazement, the patient's tumors regressed. The drug was injected into other patients with the same result. Bubbling with excitement, the research trio relayed the dramatic results to the military, but their excitement was short lived. Because of the secrecy still surrounding the US military war gas program, they were told to keep quiet. The results were not allowed to be published until three years later.

When the results were finally published in 1946, they inspired a wave of excitement. For centuries, surgery and radiation had dominated the landscape of cancer treatment, the success of which depended upon whether the cancer had spread. If it had, the utility of both radiation and the surgical knife vanished. And of course drugs were the only conceivable solution to "liquid" cancers like leukemia and lymphoma that were impossible to cut out or irradiate. The idea of drugs that could diffuse through the body, bringing the fight to cancer wherever it hid, had been a long-standing dream. The success of nitrogen mustard sparked a tantalizing possibility: maybe drugs could be developed to treat or even cure cancer. Researchers and physicians around the world were captivated by the potential.

Once the first chemotherapeutic agent was administered to lymphoma patients across the country, a new era of oncology was ushered in. The context of its birth was heavy with metaphor. The world's first chemotherapeutic agent was conceived from a substance designed to maim and break the will of enemies in a cloud of slow-moving death. Its therapeutic potential was discovered during a terrible accident in some of humanity's darkest years.

"If one reads the literature of the time, there was a real sense of excitement that perhaps drugs could cure patients with cancer," Vincent DeVita, Jr., the prominent oncologist, wrote of the first widespread use of nitrogen mustard as a chemotherapeutic agent. After the drug was widely distributed and some time had passed, the excitement proved to be premature. The remissions from nitrogen mustard turned out to be brief and incomplete. The drug was able to "soften" the typically hard nodes for only a matter of weeks. The cancer then sprang back to life, again packing the lymph nodes full of solid malignancy. It was a blow to the fragile, tantalizing hope for chemotherapy. The euphoria was followed by pessimism, and the prospect that drugs could affect the outcome for cancer patients in any meaningful way was again shrouded in uncertainty.

Nitrogen mustard works by attacking DNA itself. The nucleotides or base pairs of DNA bind through interactions called hydrogen bonds. Of all the different ways atoms can form connections, hydrogen bonds are among the weakest. They are the "soft handshake" of molecular bonds. This is important for the functionality of DNA. When a cell divides, the helical structure of DNA needs to unwind, exposing each strand individually so that it can be copied. All twenty-three chromosomal pairs replicate themselves prior to cell division, one copy for each new cell. The pliable nature of hydrogen bonds allows DNA to be dynamic, unzipping when specific genes are called to be transcribed into RNA, and then protein, or unzipping to prepare for cell division.

Nitrogen mustard works by seeking out the nucleotide guanine and locking it into a permanent handshake with its partner cytosine. This prevents DNA from being able to unzip, thus preventing cell division. Of course, nitrogen mustard is unable to distinguish a normal cell from cancerous ones, so it travels through the body indiscriminately, locking the DNA of every cell it encounters and freezing it in place, like a parking attendant putting a boot on the wheel of a car. The result of this attack is what might be expected from injecting a war gas into a patient's vein. A few hours after injection, a patient is hit with waves of nausea, followed by vomiting as the body tries to rid itself of the poison. In the weeks that follow, red blood cells, white blood cells, and platelets drop precipitously as the cell division necessary for blood production is halted by the mustard compound. Bruises begin to appear as clotting is inhibited. Anemia induces a fatigue so consuming that patients are unable to care for themselves in the most rudimentary of ways. The chance of infection greatly increases from the decimation of the immune system. As more time passes and the DNA of more cells is locked up, hair cannot grow, and it begins to fall out. The rapidly dividing cells of the gut lining are killed, resulting in uncontrolled diarrhea; black and tarry episodes result from intestinal bleeding. Patients become sterile from the poison's assault on the cells of sex organs. Mouth sores appear, and the veins used to carry the drug to the rest of the body begin to darken.

As World War II came to its conclusion, and the world began the slow process of getting back to normal, the pessimism surrounding chemotherapy and the disappointment of nitrogen mustard lifted enough to allow reconsideration. Perhaps it lifted because it had to. The uncomfortable fact was that cancer treatment had been stagnant for centuries and consisted of only two principles: remove as much as possible with surgery and treat what was left with radiation.

As infectious disease became less of a burden, progress in cancer remained nonexistent. By 1926, cancer had become the nation's second-leading cause of death. The public would not have to wait long, however. Methotrexate, discovered by Sidney Farber in 1947, was found to be capable of invoking remissions in children with leukemia, again sparking hope for a third line of treatment.

Farber was born in Buffalo, New York, in 1903. Trained as a pathologist, Farber eventually became more interested in treating patients than the lonely pursuit of examining samples in the confines of a laboratory. For Farber, what began as an interest morphed into a peculiar obsession. He became infatuated with the dream of chemotherapy, the fabled third line of cancer treatment, but like nitrogen mustard, methotrexate evoked fleeting remissions measured only in weeks. As he mulled over a strategy that might overcome the transient remissions he had a model to look to: the newly discovered power of antibiotics. The public was introduced to the exotic-sounding compounds with annual frequency: chloramphenicol in 1947, tetracycline one year later, and streptomycin the year after that. For doctors like Farber, dreaming of similar drugs for cancer, antibiotics were a beacon of hope to conquer disease. Beyond their almost magical properties, the growing arsenal of antibiotics did something else. They allowed doctors to design clinical trials and map the best way to administer them. The well-designed and well-executed trials taught physicians that there was power in combination. When the pathogen parried, they switched weapons and jousted, keeping the pathogen on its toes.

Doctors like Farber took notice. Perhaps the same strategy could be applied to cancer, and perhaps the stalemate could be broken in their favor by alternating or combining drugs. But Farber and others realized that to get combinations, they needed more drugs.

In the summer of 1946, Farber's first attempt to develop a chemotherapy drug worked in spite of himself. Learning that folic acid (folate) could treat anemia, he sloppily reasoned that because the vitamin exerted its effect on blood production, maybe it would, somehow, push the overproduction of blood in leukemia patients toward normality. But Farber soon found that his logic was exactly backward.

The vitamin was required for DNA to replicate; to give it to a leukemia patient was to pour gasoline on a fire. Once injected, the patient's cell counts exploded, violently accelerating the disease. Undeterred, Farber simply turned his line of reasoning inside out. If folic acid made leukemia worse, maybe antifolic acid would make it better. He needed a molecule that looked just enough like folic acid to trick the body into thinking it was the real thing, a molecular decoy of sorts.

Fortunately for Farber a pharmaceutical chemist named Yellapragada Subbarao in upstate New York was tinkering with ways to synthesize folate from scratch. Synthetic chemistry is as much an art form as a science. Starting with a given compound, synthetic chemists draw on experience and intuition to add, rearrange, and subtract molecular groups from the original compound until the desired product is obtained. As Subbarao worked toward his goal of folate, he generated intermediates that were similar in structure to folate but might differ in a few atoms here or there. To Subbarao, the intermediates were more or less meaningless, just a means to an end, but to Farber, they were precisely what he was looking for. One compound, methotrexate, had a molecular topology that was close enough to folate that the cell was unable to tell the difference. Even though to the cell methotrexate looked like folate, it didn't act like folate. Rather, it acted like a broken key in a lock, gumming up the process and halting the biological process required by folate, thereby halting the replication of DNA.

Like nitrogen mustard, methotrexate was far from specific. It indiscriminately prevented both cancerous cells and normal cells from dividing, but because cancer cells divided more often, it killed them with a slight preference. Like nitrogen mustard, Farber's drug was able to eke out only brief remissions, but it was enough. His discovery inspired the unbridled energy of activist and philanthropist Mary Lasker. Holding up methotrexate as an example, she urged the US Congress to initiate a national program dedicated to the discovery of more drugs. In 1955, she got her wish. The Senate Appropriations Committee allocated $5 million for the development of the Cancer Chemotherapy National Service Center (CCNSC), a program that would "change the face of cancer drug development in the world and changed the NCI and NIH irrevocably," according to DeVita, the former director of NCI.

Drugs of the same ilk followed. In 1951, Gertrude Elion, a brilliant synthetic chemist, designed a molecule to look like one of the four bases of DNA, following the same logic used for methotrexate but from a slightly different angle. If the molecule could trick the cell into thinking it was a nucleotide, then it could throw a wrench in the process of DNA replication. Like nitrogen mustard and methotrexate, Elion's drug, 6-mercaptopurine (6-MP) threw the patients into remission, and like the other drugs, it was measured only in weeks. But even if the drugs by themselves disappointed, slowly an arsenal was being built. While alone the drugs may have been weak, doctors reasoned that, like antibiotics, together they might be strong. But one thing was different about chemotherapy drugs when compared to antibiotics. There was no hiding the fact that they were blunt, indiscriminate poisons. To use them in combination, as antibiotics were used, might improve the outcome, but it might also double or triple the toxicity, killing the patients before they could get better.

Ying and Yang

It took the blend of boldness and caution to move the idea of combining the new drugs into patients. In the spring of 1955, the serendipitous collision of audacious courage and thoughtful caution occurred at NCI.

Emil Freireich was bold, confident, and flamboyant, while his counterpart, Emil Frei, was cautious, soft spoken and thoughtful—one the yin, the other the yang. Throughout his career, Frei did things like dressing up like Big Bird or Darth Vader for the sick kids. Siddhartha Mukherjee described Frei making rounds on a pediatric oncology ward: "He was charming, soft spoken and careful. To watch him manage critically ill children and their testy, nervous parents was to watch a champion swimmer glide through water—so adept in the art that he made artistry vanish."

His partner, Freireich, was a buzz saw. Described as having a "volcanic" temper, Freireich was fired seven times over the course of his career. He came from a harsh beginning. His father committed suicide after the 1929 stock market crash, and his family was cast into abject poverty. Where Frei came from a family of artists, Freireich described his childhood by saying, "I'd never seen a ballet. I'd never seen a play. Outside of our little TV that my mother purchased, I had no education to speak of. There was no literature, no art. No music, no dance, no nothing. It was just food. And not getting killed or beaten up. I was pretty raw."

As different as they were, together, they provided a union of checks and balances needed to move forward with combinational chemotherapy. When Freireich lost his temper or pushed too hard, Frei gently reeled him in. Many on the periphery were questioning the concept of toxic chemotherapy, let alone combinations of the drugs. Even single drugs, if pushed too far, devastated the patients. Freireich learned this the hard way with a drug called vincristine. "Of the first fourteen children we treated, one or two actually died. Their brains were totally fried." Most declared it "inhumane" to drip poison into the veins of patients, so if they were to proceed, they would have to tread lightly. But to surpass the hiccough-type responses produced by single drugs, they would have to use the power of combination, they would have to push boundaries.

During the winter of 1957, the duo was finally given permission to treat children with leukemia with a combination of two drugs, Farber's methotrexate combined with 6-MP. The study also included two additional arms where patients were given one drug each. The study was designed with one goal: to determine whether chemotherapy drugs were more powerful when used in combination. When the results were tallied, the difference was striking. Given alone, the drugs produced response rates between 15 and 20 percent. Combined, the responses were much better. Although the combination of drugs was extremely toxic, riding on a knife's edge of tolerability, it boosted remission rates by more than 45 percent. Now it was known that combining chemotherapy drugs improved the outcome of patients. As learned from antibiotics, the one-two punch flanked the problem of drug resistance. The results set the stage moving forward, but the path was not without friction.

As the fledgling field of cancer chemotherapy was taking shape, it galvanized doctors into opposing camps. One camp wanted to push forward, and the other felt that it came at too high a price. Even though patients faced an invariably fatal disease, some felt that to put them through hell for what time they had left was morally reprehensible. Depending on a doctor's disposition, all it took was a peek in the treatment rooms as doctors walked through the leukemia ward at the NCI hospital to put them in one camp or the other. Max Wintrope, the oncologist, said, "These drugs cause more harm than good, because they just prolong the agony. The patients all die anyway." Freireich didn't see it that way; in fact, he saw the opposite. "My feeling was I'll try it. Why not? They're going to die anyway." The leukemia ward at the hospitals contained ashen-faced kids huddled over buckets—anemic zombies of sorts. To label what was happening in the name of experimentation as "cruel" and "insane," as many did, may have been the easy way out. Others pointed out that the kids had no other options. They had a disease that sentenced them to death. Even so, it took a certain individual to intentionally put them through chemotherapeutic hell. Many would have no part of it and were quick to judge those who were doing so.

As they trudged forward, below the surface, guiding principles were developed. As far back as the thirties, a scientist documented that the transfer of a single leukemia cell was sufficient to kill a mouse. The resounding message was that to rid a patient of cancer meant leaving not a single cell behind. The fact that a single cell was enough to reignite malignancy was daunting considering that a dose of chemotherapy didn't kill a specific number of cells but a fraction of the overall burden. The implication was obvious: the longer chemotherapy could be drawn out, the more likely the probability of extinguishing the disease down to the very last cell and, by extension, the more likely that the patient would be cured. The optimists still believed there was a chance that real cures could be realized for a least a fraction of the children with leukemia.

In the early sixties a creative hunch began brewing in Freireich's mind. He reasoned that because certain drugs killed cancer cells by different mechanisms, the toxicity would be diluted instead of being additive. Every doctor knew that dose determined toxicity. If someone stacked too many quarters in one spot on a sheet of paper, it would eventually rip through, but what if the quarters were stacked on different spots? The paper could hold substantially more weight by spreading the weight out.

Freireich reasoned that the same principle might work when combining drugs—the toxicity might be spread out. He approached Frei with his logic. They already knew that combining drugs increased the capacity to wipe out cancer cells. Months of intense discussion culminated in a bold strategic regimen that combined four drugs: vincristine, amethopterin, mercaptopurine, and prednisone, a regimen given the acronym VAMP. When they presented their plan at a national meeting for blood cancers, it evoked gasps from the audience. Many, including Farber, disagreed with the approach, favoring a rotation with single drugs administered one at a time. It was far from clear whether the poisonous cocktail would be too much for the sick children, killing more than helping. There was a lot riding on Freireich's hunch. It took Frei's diplomatic touch to convince others that the four-drug regimen was worth a try, but in the end, they were given the green light to go ahead with VAMP.

When the trial was launched in 1961, it appeared that those who said VAMP was insane had the correct impulse. The four-drug combination devastated the children's cell counts, plunging the children to the point where they were left hanging by a thread. Frei and Freireich expected devastating side effects. Knowing full well the delicate nature of the trial, the doctors did everything they could to limp the children through to the end. If the children began to die, it would be an enormous blow for everyone involved. Platelet transfusions were given to prevent bleeding, combinations of new and old antibiotics were given to prevent infection. For three anxious weeks, everybody— including NCI staff, who had taken a big risk in approving the trial in the first place—watched with bated breath.

When the finish line finally arrived, and the dust settled, the tremendous suffering and anxiety had a payoff. As the kids' pummeled bone marrow slowly recovered, again trickling out a steady stream of blood cells, one thing was different. The grossly distorted leukemia cells that once flowed alongside the normal cells were conspicuously absent. It was a huge victory for the NCI and the two Emils. As striking as the remissions were, they would have to prove durable. The question was whether the regimen eradicated all the leukemia cells, curing the children's disease, or whether there were cells yet in hiding, buying time before continuing their relentless march. Only time would tell.

MOPP

It was clear which camp Vincent DeVita fell into when he joined NCI in 1963. The brash New Yorker, whose mother often found him dissecting frogs on the front steps of their Yonkers home when he was a boy, found himself "suddenly surrounded by these maniacs doing cancer research." The hard-charging and superheated atmosphere created by Frei and Freireich "infected" DeVita, and the cardiologist was hypnotically drawn into their controversial club.

The field of medical oncology didn't exist. It was being forged, but to join the inner circle, DeVita found there was a price to pay. Colleagues watching from the sidelines labeled Frei, Freireich, and DeVita the "lunatic fringe"—they were confronted with sideways looks, scoffs, or open hostility. Other doctors referred to the drugs they were using simply as "poison." Many felt that they were not pioneering, brave, or bold—instead viewing them as unethical, inhumane, and barbaric. DeVita said, "It took plain old courage to be a chemotherapist in the 1960s." Operating under such a banner of skepticism and derision, he knew that the burden of proof was heavy. They would have to unequivocally prove that chemotherapy did more good than harm.

Buoyed by the initial remissions from the VAMP trial, DeVita set out to prove the viability of the new approach. To do this he knew that he would need to tackle another cancer, establishing that the approach could be applied outward. He chose Hodgkin's disease, an invariably fatal but rare form of lymphoma. Hodgkin's tended to strike preferentially by age (in young adulthood or after the age of fifty-five). It tended to present in a predictable pattern, marching from one lymph node to the next in a choreographed sequence. Others had shown that localized disease could be successfully felled by radiation, but systemic disease had no other treatment options, making it a good candidate for chemotherapy.

DeVita chose a regime mirroring that of VAMP, a four-drug combination consisting of nitrogen mustard, Oncovin (the brand name for vincristine), procarbazine, and prednisone (MOPP), a swirling mixture of the controversial new treatment paradigm. He recalled that when they presented the idea to NCI, the proposal was met with "fierce" resistance, again forcing Frei to step in and gently and diplomatically overrule the critics.

Beginning in 1964, the victims of advanced Hodgkin's began to sign up to receive DeVita's new protocol. Forty-three patients received MOPP from kids not yet teenagers, to old men, and every age in-between. Like VAMP, MOPP was mapping the undiscovered country of cancer therapy, but it was also exploring a new frontier of side effects. Many thought that the blunt approach was premature and that understanding of a disease should come first, with rational therapies to follow. DeVita's approach was the opposite. Forged from the simple crucible of trial and error, therapy, he reasoned, could precede understanding. He wasn't going to wait for basic science to catch up.

As expected, MOPP drove patients into a haze of debilitating nausea that struck in vicious and unpredictable waves. The immune system was destroyed, leaving them exposed to a swath of pathogens from the rare and exotic to the commonplace. Every effort was made to keep them from getting sick, but microbes often found their way into their defenseless bodies, sickening them with pneumonia and other illnesses. In addition to common side effects like hair loss and vomiting, unanticipated ones like sterility in both men and women were created. Like VAMP, once the limits of tolerability and morality were stretched to the snapping point, the payoff phase eclipsed the ugliness. The swollen nodes disappeared. The patients slowly recovered, their hair grew back, they could keep food down, and health was restored.

Chemotherapy was a new form of healing that was designed to tear the body down and then allow it to heal. The hope was that the distorted cancer cells, wherever they came from, were unable to make the journey back. It was like burning down a house to rid it of rats, hoping, in the end, that it could still be rebuilt. Whatever invisible event conspired to spark Hodgkin's genesis didn't matter. For the moment, the cancer was gone.

In the fall of 1963, just a few years after the last child was treated with VAMP, the cautious optimism that permeated the hallways of the cancer ward suffered a devastating blow. The striking remissions achieved from the VAMP trial proved to not be as enduring as hoped. One by one, Frei and Freireich's children returned to the clinic with a cadre of neurological complaints. One child had a seizure, another had a strange tingling sensation, and another had persistent headaches. The optimism they allowed to seep in was replaced by a heavy stillness. Freireich suspected that these weren't symptoms that would go away. Cerebrospinal fluid was extracted through spinal taps for analysis. What they found crushed any remaining hope. Inside the murky fluid was the culprit: leukemia cells. VAMP had ridded the bone marrow and lymph nodes of leukemia, but the cancer took asylum in the body's protected neurological embassy. It went to the one place it couldn't be followed. All it took was a few cells to squeeze through the blood-brain barrier, the cellular seal that protected the brain from environmental toxins. Hidden, the colonialist cancer cells began new rounds of growth, and the children felt the symptoms presented to Frei and Freireich: blurred vision, headaches, and weird tingles. As the growth arc continued, the children fell into comas followed quickly by death.

Frei and Freireich had to watch helplessly as the children they had poured every fiber of their being into helping, kids whose lives were emotionally intertwined with their own, spiraled to their deaths as the cancer exploded within the safety of the brain. The bold enthusiasm the doctors were known for was, in a matter of a few months, completely deflated. The devastation of the trial they had pinned so much hope on was too much to take. The voices of all the skeptics who openly questioned why they were putting the children thorough such hell now held a poignant sting. In the winter of 1963, Frei left NCI, and Freireich soon followed.

It would be more than a decade before Varmus and Bishop snapped together the loose ends describing the molecular details thought to turn a cell cancerous, providing a blueprint for therapeutic design. Until then, the only way forward was to continue the path cut by Frei, Freireich, and DeVita. Even if doctors knew little of the cancer cell's nature, they were learning how it behaved on the battlefield.

With Frei and Freireich out of the picture, a new soldier needed to take over where they left off. As before, it would take a maverick, someone capable of ignoring detractors. As VAMP trailed off into oblivion, Donald Pinkel, a Navy doctor, showed up at NIH to pick up the pieces of the broken trial, reorganize them, and try again.

Total Therapy

Born in Buffalo, New York, in 1926, Pinkel was the fifth of seven children born to his German-American father and Irish-Canadian mother. "Each was raised by impoverished widows, left school early and knew hardship," he said. After graduating from medical school at the University of Buffalo in 1951, like his parents, he also found himself on the receiving end of hardship when he contracted polio while caring for sick children at the US Army Hospital in Fort Devens, Massachusetts, in 1954.

> *I thought I was immune to it. We had big epidemics in Buffalo in the 1950s, and I took care of hundreds of children with polio. But at Fort Devens I happened to be over-tired; I was staying up a lot with sick children and I was the only pediatrician. I came down with it worse than any of my patients. While hospitalized at Fort Devens, my respiratory function went down to a small fraction. I remember going to sleep one night and thinking, "Well, this is it. I'm not going to wake up."*

Pinkel fought back, drawing inspiration from something his high school football coach had told him long ago: "Never run away from a fight. The farther you run, the more difficult it will be to fight back." He eventually recovered but suffered from partial paralysis. In 1962, he opened St. Jude Children's Research Hospital in Memphis and turned his focus to acute lymphoblastic leukemia.

He again tapped his fighting spirit as he begin to engineer a new regimen to combat Acute lymphoblastic leukemia (ALL), a regimen that would fight the disease with a vicious ferocity that nobody dreamed possible. Because of the VAMP trial, he knew where the cancer cells were hiding, just beyond the fragile blood-brain barrier in the cerebrospinal fluid.

This time he injected drugs directly into the safe haven, removing the reason for VAMP's failure. To extinguish the possibility that even a single cancer cell survived the assault, he dosed the brain with radiation, just to make absolutely sure. Reasoning that VAMP alone might be too soft of an approach, he proposed combinations of combinations, scrambling up to eight different drugs, attacking the cancer from every conceivable direction. And again, to remove any possibility of a single surviving cell, he stretched the duration of the treatment from months into years. He called the approach "Total Therapy," reflective of its design to not leave a single cancer cell behind. His radical approach was timed perfectly. The attitude surrounding chemotherapy was much more permissive because of the success of DeVita's MOPP trial. But even in a more permissive environment, Pinkel's Total Therapy stood out. "Most people thought we were nuts," he said.

As he went to recruit doctors for the trial, most refused once they read the extreme protocol. He was left with a handful of doctors who shared his enthusiasm. Even though on paper the protocol was long and exhaustively precise, the logic of Total Therapy was simple. Without a clear understanding of the disease, and with only certain weapons available, if they didn't beat the cancer the first time, then pushing harder was the only option.

When the survivor data was tallied, Pinkel and DeVita were transformed from ethical pariahs to heroes. Eighty percent of Pinkel's kids were estimated to be cured. DeVita was able to cure 60 percent of his patients with Hodgkin's disease. The news of the cure rate achieved by the bold administration of combinations of drugs was celebrated. Parties were thrown, awards were given, and there was a feeling that a new era of cancer therapy had been born. "By the end of the 1960s, the missing link of the chemotherapy program had been forged, and it was now clear that anticancer drugs could cure cancer," DeVita wrote.

As the accomplishments were celebrated on television and in newspapers and magazines everywhere, young doctors were learning by example. Too much caution could avert real advance in medicine. It was a fine line, but there were rewards for being the one brave enough to push boundaries, even in the face of opposition. It was a lesson that, in the years ahead, would have to be unlearned as a new generation applied the approach to more difficult forms of cancer. And the logic to "push harder" would kill the patient before killing the cancer.

"That Son of a Bitch"

Two days before Christmas in 1971, President Richard Nixon took the podium and, in a speech before the US Congress, declared war against cancer. There was an undeniable hubris in his facial expression and tone of voice and the content of the declaration. America had emerged from Thomas Hobbes's state of helplessness against the forces of nature with spectacular speed. We could do anything. Two years prior, we put a man on the moon. We battled back infectious disease with new drugs and hygienic practices. Once we understood the pathogenic mechanism, treatment and prevention rapidly followed.

The success of combinatorial chemotherapy contributed to the feeling that no challenge was insurmountable if Americans put their hearts into it. It was widely believed that it would be only a matter of years before a general cure for cancer was discovered. It was simply a matter of getting the right combination and dose of drugs. With coffers buoyed by Nixon's National Cancer Act, NIH pushed as hard as it could with the weapons it had. With targeted therapy still in its infancy, this meant continuing the same toxic, indiscriminate, and blunt war. MOPP, VAMP, and Pinkel's Total Therapy established the foundation of chemotherapeutic logic: combine drugs, up the dose, hit first, and hit hard. The medical slang for cancer treatment, "slash and burn" (surgery and radiation) now had a third component: "slash, burn, and poison."

NCI turned into a drug-screening factory. The Developmental Therapeutics Program (DTP) budget swelled to $68 million and transformed into a drug-screening juggernaut, churning through three million mice and screening forty thousand drugs annually. The process spun off an industry of oncological pharmaceuticals once it was proven the drugs could be prescribed and a profit could be realized. Even though it had grown immensely, cancer drug development was still guided by the most rudimentary of logic: find the agents that inhibited cell division. Other indiscriminate poisons came out of the program. Cisplatin was one of the more exciting drugs put into trials. It operated with the same mechanism as its cousin, nitrogen mustard, locking strands of DNA together and rendering replication impossible. Like its cousin, it was also discovered by accident (it was noticed for its ability to inhibit the growth of bacteria suspended in liquid).

Throughout the seventies, the clinical mission continued but with many more resources and, because of the success of MOPP and Total Therapy, a new sense of bravado. The budget available for a single branch of clinical trials swelled from $9 million in 1972 to $119 million in 1980. Large-scale, multi-institutional trials began in earnest. The previous successes, and taxpayer support, infused cancer wards with an aura of optimism. "Did we believe we were going to cure cancer with all these chemicals? Absolutely we did," George Canellos, a colleague of DeVita, said. "We spoke of curing cancer as if it was almost a given."

A seemingly unending supply of new patients provided a fresh canvas for experimentation with new drugs, combinations of existing drugs, or combinations of old with new. The doctors bombarded patients, sending them to the brink of death, brought them back, and bombarded them again. The effort to care for each patient to the end—patting heads, wiping brows, and considering every detail that would make the patient more comfortable—may have been an attempt to sanitize what NCI clinics had morphed into: trial and error on a massive scale.

In the background, as the basic science of cancer research trudged forward, others couldn't help commenting on the indiscriminate experimentation. James Watson was against the clinical cancer centers. He argued the funds should go toward "pure cancer research," basic science and investigation that would reveal the fundamental nature of cancer. No one listened, and the institute continued its mission of attacking cancer with carpet bombs rather than guided missiles. Watson's reward for openly disagreeing was to be kicked off the advisory board after only two years. He watched from the sidelines as toxic cocktails were dripped into the veins of patients in the name of research. In 1977, as perhaps the apex of unenlightened boldness was reached, he remarked on the course of the cancer effort, "We shall so poison the atmosphere of the first act that no one of decency shall want to see the play through to the end."

Cisplatin became so popular that it became known as the "penicillin" of cancer. With the yellow toxin came a virulence of nausea not seen before—on average, patients taking cisplatin vomited once every hour they were awake. As the colorful chemicals dripped into the patients, a spectrum of side effects ensued that left no organ or cell unscathed. Kidneys were put into failure, hearts were damaged, lungs and skin were scarred and burnt, hearing was lost, septic shock was induced, and immune systems were devastated. Many patients even died outright from the trials. "Chemotherapy is just medieval. It's such a blunt instrument. We're going to look back on it like we do the dark ages," physician and author Eric Topol said.

The director of NCI encouraged the doctors to expand the chemotherapeutic-paradigm outward to "solid" cancers, the ruthless forms that were responsible for 95 percent of all cancer deaths. The shift garnered some initial success when a doctor named Lawrence Einhorn treated testicular cancer with the combination of bleomycin, vinblastine, and cisplatin (BVP). With the new regimen, Einhorn moved the cure rate from 10 percent to 85 percent, a colossal achievement, but testicular cancer proved to be the weakest of the lot. When doctors moved to other solid cancers, the drugs proved ineffectual. Even as they tried different combinations and upped the dose, they were able to beat the cancer back for weeks or months at best. It seemed as though they had exhausted the utility of the drugs.

The first act of chemotherapy had hit a wall. It was lucky that the drugs achieved what they did considering that they were largely discovered by accident or identified through simple screening, guided by the most rudimentary of principles. Cytotoxic chemotherapy, without question, would one day be looked back on by future physicians as a terribly primitive episode in medical history, similar to how we look back today at medieval medical practices. For now, toxic chemotherapy was inextricably intertwined with cancer, shaping the way we viewed the disease. The nature of chemotherapy framed the restoration of health as a fight or a battle. Someone with cancer was at "war" with the disease. Abraham Verghese, professor for the theory and practice of medicine at Stanford University Medical School, said,

> In America, we have always taken it as an article of faith that we "battle" cancer; we attack it with knives, we poison it with chemotherapy or we blast it with radiation. If we are fortunate, we "beat" the cancer. If not, we are posthumously praised for having "succumbed after a long battle."

As NIH's clinical mission continued into the 1980s, it encountered a stumbling block. The statisticians did something many labeled outrageous: they looked closely at the numbers. Numbers cut through the swath of biases. People may disagree on a number of issues, but numbers don't lie; like it or not, raw data simply *is*. But not this time. With so much money, careers, and emotion invested into NCI's cancer drug development, the overall statistics became the center of a heated controversy. Over a decade into the war against cancer, it was time to objectively assess the results.

Chemotherapy and the Gates of Hell

When the bio-statisticians released their findings in 1986, they were instantly demonized. "Reprehensible," DeVita said of "Progress in Cancer?" published in *The New England Journal of Medicine*. The analysis didn't come from a dubious source. It came from a Yale-educated physician named John Bailer, who earned a PhD in biostatistics and then went to work at NCI—one of their own. And Bailer and his colleagues weren't doing anything worth demonizing. They were simply counting and doing their job. A hard look at the numbers told the story.

The generous assumption was that three thousand lives were saved by the advance made in childhood leukemia, Hodgkin's disease, testicular cancer, Burkett's lymphoma, and a few other rare cancers. Adding in the lives saved by adjunctive chemotherapy and preventative measures like Pap smears and mammograms brought the total lives saved to forty thousand a year. In 1985, a million people were diagnosed with cancer. The math revealed that all efforts combined since the "war on cancer" began saved 4 percent of those diagnosed with cancer. Of course, to the individuals within the 4 percent, the war was an unmitigated success—it was impossible to diminish any life saved.

As Bailer dug further, he focused on the only number that mattered: the raw death rate, the sheer body count. The raw death rate intrinsically had all bias removed, it alone told the real story. And it told it from all angles. By counting the bodies left on the "battlefield," every aspect of the war on cancer was included from new cases (a number reflecting how "carcinogenic" our lifestyles were) to the number of people saved by *all* medical intervention.

The analysis read like this: since 1950, death by cancer *had increased by 9 percent*. The influence of lifestyle, and how carcinogenic we had made our world, dwarfed every effort made to combat cancer (probably largely attributed to the increase in smoking rates in the 1950s). Looking at the only yardstick that mattered, we were losing the war, or at the least our focus was dead wrong. Prevention clearly mattered more than desperately trying to find cures. Unable to argue with the math, many invested in the chemotherapeutic-cause attacked Bailer personally. The president of the American Society of Clinical Oncology (ASCO) called Bailer "the great naysayer of our time." According to Bailer, others simply referred to him as "that son of a bitch."

Years later, survival data revealed another surprise. Beyond the debilitating side effects, there was an additional price to pay for the massive doses of toxins injected into the sick children. Decades later, *The New England Journal of Medicine* published follow-up data:

> *In addition to sharply increased risk of heart attack and stroke, the children who were successfully treated for Hodgkin's disease are 18 times more likely later to develop secondary malignant tumors. Girls face a 35 percent chance of developing breast cancer by the time they are 40—which is 75 times greater than the average. The risk of leukemia increased markedly four years after the ending of successful treatment, and reached a plateau after 14 years, but the risk of developing solid tumors remained high and approached 30 percent at 30 years.*

The sixties and seventies were known for the unenlightened crusade against cancer using a handful of systemic toxins, but that was about to change. With Varmus and Bishop establishing the origin of cancer in 1976, researchers now had a road map. They could now begin to move away from the indiscriminate poisons of the past and approach cancer rationally. The cancer-causing protein products of oncogenes were foreign to the cell. They were the functional difference between normal cells and cancer cells, and most importantly, they were targets. "Time and time again, several different lines of inquiry into proto-oncogenes have converged on the same junction box (of cellular circuitry) it seems we may have more of the circuitry of the cell in our view than previously could have hoped. The cell is not infinitely complex. The cell can be understood," Bishop said during a 1989 Nobel lecture. With understanding would come targeted therapies designed to specifically kill cancer cells nontoxically while sparing healthy cells. "Pharmaceutical chemists may be able to invent ways to interdict the action of oncogene products," Bishop said optimistically.

In 1983, Robert Weinberg of MIT, one of the most highly esteemed cancer researchers, said, "The major details of carcinogenesis should be largely worked out by the end of this decade." Most thought that the promised targeted drugs would be quick to follow. As the 1990s began, DeVita said, "Chemotherapy has, in fact, transitioned to the age of targeted therapy."

Part 3

Breakthroughs and Disappointments

Into the Dustbin of History

When Warburg died in 1970, his theory on the origin of cancer was all but forgotten. If any flicker of it remained, most considered it extinguished when one of the world's most prominent cancer researchers, Sidney Weinhouse, wrote a review in 1976 titled, "The Warburg Hypothesis Fifty Years Later." He systematically dismantled Warburg's contention that cancer originated from damage to the cells' respiratory capacity. "Despite massive efforts during the half-century following the Warburg proposal to find some alteration of function or structure of mitochondria, that might conceivably give some measure of support to the Warburg hypothesis, no substantial evidence has been found," wrote Weinhouse. It smacked of an intellectual coup—the young guard unceremoniously overthrowing the old guard and relegating antiquated ideas into the dustbin of history. "The whole conception of cancer initiation or survival by 'faulty' respiration and high glycolysis seems too simplistic for serious consideration," Weinhouse said.

Breakthroughs and Disappointments

Though an iconic member of one of science's most decorated fraternities in a golden era of science, Warburg had his theory on the origin of cancer slain and buried. Weinhouse put the final nail in the coffin the same year that Varmus and Bishop established mutations to DNA as the singular and undisputed origin of cancer. Warburg's theory joined the list of disproven theories, ideas that grew like branches from the tree of knowledge only to die and fall off.

Five years after Weinhouse's scathing review, in 1981, Hans Krebs, Warburg's former student, friend, and fellow Nobel laureate, wrote a biography of Warburg titled *Otto Warburg: Cell Physiologist, Biochemist, and Eccentric*, so that his spectacular career would not be forgotten. Even to Krebs, for Warburg, cancer research may have been the only blemish on what was an otherwise outstanding career. Krebs wrote this of the speech Warburg gave at the Lindau meeting four years before his death:

He still showed a clear, logical, and forceful style but the balance of his judgment, in the view of most experts, is at fault. His sweeping generalizations spring from gross simplification. The partial replacement of respiration by glycolysis is only one of many characteristics which distinguish cancer cells from normal cells. Warburg neglected the fundamental biochemical aspect of the cancer problem, that of the mechanisms which are responsible for the controlled growth of normal cells and which are lost or disturbed in the cancer cell. No doubt, the differences in energy metabolism discovered by Warburg are important, but however important; they are at the level of the biochemical organization of the cell, not deep enough to touch the heart of the cancer problem, the uncontrolled growth. Warburg's "primary cause of cancer"— may be a symptom of the primary cause, but is not the primary cause itself. The primary cause is to be expected at the level of

*the control of the gene expression, the minutiae of which are
unknown though some of the principals involved are understood.*

A Flickering Ember

With all eyes fixed on DNA, nobody noticed that an ember of Warburg's theory still burned, one that would be nurtured and methodically brought back to life.

Warburg was able to grossly describe what he believed to be the fundamental alteration in cancer cells: they fermented glucose in the presence of oxygen. But Warburg failed to discover *why* or *how* cancer cells exhibited the Warburg effect. After Varmus and Bishop's discovery of the cellular origin of viral oncogenes in 1976—and with Warburg thoroughly discredited—it was not an exaggeration to say that no one except Pete Pedersen of Johns Hopkins considered the metabolism to be at the "heart" of the cancer problem. The work he did while nobody was paying attention served as scaffolding for future researchers to climb as decades passed and they begin to realize that the metabolism of cancer held a missing piece to a puzzle that genetics had not been able to solve.

Born in 1939, Pedersen is well over six feet tall with rangy limbs, a steady gaze, a firm handshake, and a soft voice with locutions reminiscent of old Western actors. He doesn't fit the stereotype of an East Coast intellectual, but nothing of Pedersen fits a stereotypical mold.

Pedersen's father, the son of Danish immigrants, migrated from Wisconsin to Oklahoma in the late 1930s, thinking that the cheap land would open up opportunities. Once he got there, he discovered why the land was so cheap. It was blowing away as the dust bowl era took hold. About the same time, Pedersen's mother, of part Cherokee heritage, moved from Arkansas to Oklahoma for a secretarial job. The two met, married, and had three boys and a girl. The family was a unique American amalgam, a melding of immigrant with indigenous. He called his heritage a hybrid of *The Grapes of Wrath* and the Trail of Tears. When he was a boy, they moved to Catoosa, Oklahoma, a town on the outskirts of Tulsa. Struggling to find work, his father eventually found a job as a traveling salesman. When World War II broke out, his father then landed a job at the Douglas Aircraft Company in Tulsa. To supplement the family's income, his father began a strawberry farm, and as a young man, Pedersen spent long hours in the fields.

The family began to enjoy some modest prosperity. As early as Pedersen could remember, his mother's true love was chemistry. She had taken college courses in Arkansas before moving to Oklahoma. "But in those days, as a woman, she could not get any other position." She watched as her older brother, Leo Shin, obtained a degree in chemistry from the University of Arkansas. He eventually became the head of the biochemistry branch of naval research in Washington, DC, in 1952, and Pedersen remembered his mother talking a lot about her older brother and chemistry. The kids entered high school, and chemistry was not on the curriculum of the small Indian school. "My mother was determined to bring chemistry to the school," Pedersen said. She petitioned the school board and succeeded, but there was no one to teach it. "So my brother, the math teacher, and I, read a chemistry text book, bought some chemicals, and began to have a great time making mixtures that stunk up the whole school."

When their kids graduated from high school, the only college the parents could afford was a small Catholic college that had opened in Tulsa. There Pedersen and his brother encountered a nun who shared their love of chemistry, inspiring them to work after hours. He and his older brother soon realized that if they were going to succeed in the world of chemistry, they would have to go to a larger university. "Somehow we managed to get accepted to the University of Tulsa and paid for it by working late hours and weekends at separate Safeway supermarkets," Pedersen said. He and his brother graduated from the University of Tulsa with degrees in chemistry. Both followed in their mother's and uncle's footsteps and went to the University of Arkansas where Pedersen received a PhD in biochemistry, and his brother, Lee, received a PhD in theoretical chemistry.

Over the years Pedersen became increasingly interested in cancer. He knew at some point in his future he wanted to enter the field of cancer research. "I knew it was a big problem, many people I had known had died from it, and I wanted to see if I could make any progress in understanding it or treating it," he said. Upon his arrival at Johns Hopkins School of Medicine in Baltimore for postdoctoral work in 1964, Pedersen, the farm kid who went to a tiny Indian school with a graduating class of twenty-three, was intimidated, but he noticed that he had an advantage. "When you come to a place like Hopkins, and you have to compete with all these brilliant people, I realized I was way ahead of them, not because I was smarter, but because I could out work all of them," he said.

The timing was perfect. He went to work for the famous biochemist Albert Lehninger, a giant in the field of energy metabolism. In 1948, along with his student Eugene Kennedy, Lehninger discovered that mitochondria were the site of the cells' energy production, igniting an explosion in the understanding of cellular energetics. "Lehninger was a wonderful mentor," said Pedersen. "He often spoke of Warburg and knew Warburg personally." The serendipitous collision with the leading biochemist and his connection to Warburg created the perfect atmosphere for a young biochemist interested in cancer. Pedersen said, "It was like a passing of the baton, from Warburg to me, through Lehninger."

But the era of great biochemists, especially those studying cancer, was essentially over. If Pedersen was to continue the line, he would have to go it alone. When Lehninger died in 1986, Pedersen was one of the final links to Warburg. He was left as one of the few shouldering the notion that the answer to cancer lay in metabolism.

His laboratory worked in isolation, engulfed by some of America's most prestigious professors and students, all of them considering the metabolism of cancer a relic of the past, largely irrelevant, and Pedersen a throwback from a different era. The hard-working Oklahoman stayed true to his scientific lineage and the vision of his predecessors. Pedersen wrote,

> *I felt almost alone in considering energy metabolism as important to the cancer problem. I even remember one of my colleagues, an expert in DNA technology, dumping Lehninger's "Warburg Flasks" in the trash as relics of a bygone era in cancer research. Fortunately for him, Lehninger was no longer the department chair, and fortunately for me, I salvaged many of these flasks and am now glad I did.*

Nevertheless, he soldiered on. His persistence led to a series of important discoveries that coalesced into a larger image, one in which Warburg had painted the first brush stroke. Warburg pinned the origin of cancer on "injured respiration," but he lacked the experimental technology to closely study the mitochondria of cancer cells, structures he called *grana*. With the help of his mentor, Lehninger, and emerging technologies, Pedersen was able to look directly at the mitochondria of the cancer cell and set off to determine if, as Warburg guessed, they were dysfunctional.

Shortly after arriving at Johns Hopkins, Pedersen read about a researcher who had developed strains of rats harboring cancerous tumors that grew at different rates. This sparked his interest. "Some would grow very fast, killing the animal in a matter of weeks. Others would grow very slowly, taking almost a year to kill the animals. And others were in the middle," he said. The different rates of tumor growth raised an important question. What metabolic difference caused some to grow slowly and others to grow fast? The rats were developed by Harold Morris at NCI, a short drive from Johns Hopkins.

Pedersen and a technician, Joanne Hullihen, drove to NCI to meet Morris and his rats. "He was a nice guy, he gave us a number of his rats to work with." Pedersen and Hullihen loaded up the rats and drove back to Johns Hopkins.

Back in his lab Pedersen began investigating the biochemistry of the rat's tumors, and he discovered a powerful correlation. Critically, *the faster a tumor grew, and the more aggressive it was—the lower the overall number of mitochondria, and the more it fermented glucose.* He thought this counterintuitive fact revealed something fundamental about the nature of the cancer cell. He knew this correlation couldn't exist in a vacuum, and it *had* to have some significance. "That's when I began to go back and reinvestigate all this business about Warburg."

He began compiling evidence showing how injured the cancer cell's ability to respire was. Simply counting the number of mitochondria compared to normal cells provided direct evidence. Numbers alone revealed that the cancer cells had a reduced ability to respire. In every experiment, he counted the same thing: the tumor cells that exhibited a robust "Warburg effect" and grew the fastest invariably retained about 50 percent of the mitochondria compared to normal tissue matched cells. Here was a quantitative explanation for Warburg's hypothesis that cancer stemmed from insufficient respiration. It was no longer a guess, the numbers proved it.

As Pedersen dug deeper, he found that the mitochondria from cancer cells that grew the fastest were rife with a spectrum of structural abnormalities. They were smaller, less robust, cup shaped, dumbbell shaped, missing important internal membranes, and had numerous abnormalities in their protein and lipid content. Again, in biology, structure equaled function. Pedersen irrefutably showed that the mitochondria of cancer cells were structurally altered almost everywhere he looked.

By 1978, he had a compiled a massive collection of evidence showing the extent of the deficiency and/or damage to the mitochondria, and by extension, to the respiratory capacity of the cancer cell. He was resurrecting Warburg's discarded theory, but it was only two years after Varmus and Bishop sent cancer researchers off hunting oncogenes. Nobody cared about Warburg's stodgy theory, but Pedersen never questioned himself. "I knew I was right; the data didn't lie." Nevertheless, he couldn't help but be perplexed by the degree of disinterest.

In 1978, he decided that it was time to publish his findings in a massive review of the cancer cell's defective metabolism. He began the review with this question:

Despite the fact that mitochondria occupy 15–50 percent of the cytoplasmic volume of most animal cells and participate in more metabolic functions than any other organelle in the cell, it seems fair to state that cancer research, and consequently funding for it, has been directed away from mitochondrial studies in the past decade. The new student of cancer biology and biochemistry may ask "Why?"

With markedly reduced numbers and structurally distorted mitochondria, there appeared no way that cancer cells could generate sufficient energy to survive through respiration alone as Weinhouse had said they could. Having established the reason that cancer cells must generate energy by fermentation (to compensate for their missing and damaged mitochondria), Pedersen set out to discover how cancer cells ramped up fermentation. The missing and damaged mitochondria were the *why* of the Warburg effect. Pedersen wanted to discover the *how* of the Warburg effect.

In 1977, seven years after Warburg's death, Pedersen and a South American graduate student, Ernesto Bustamante, made a profound discovery. They discovered the single molecular alteration in the cell responsible for the increased fermentation that Warburg measured. The mundane title of the paper, "High Aerobic Glycolysis of Rat Hepatoma Cells in Culture: Role of Mitochondrial Hexokinase," eclipsed the vast implications of its content. "That was an important finding," the perpetually understated Pedersen said. The discovery showed why the "gas pedal" controlling fermentation was stuck to the floor in cancer cells. Perhaps more importantly, it represented a pivotal therapeutic target that was present in virtually all cancers.

Some common themes are pervasive to all forms of life. Just like all forms of life use DNA as a blueprint of instructive code, life uses a single molecule, adenosine triphosphate (ATP) as a universal carrier of metabolic energy. ATP is used in the same way that money is used as a common intermediary for transactions within an economy. ATP is the common currency of energy. The energy carried within ATP lay in a single, high-energy phosphate bond located at the end of a string of three phosphates dangling from the center. The energy released from the cleaving of this single bond is captured and redirected, facilitating movement and the myriad unseen chemical reactions that cells continuously engage in. (As you move your eyes along the words of this sentence, ATP is spent to pull one muscle fiber along another, like a person pulling a rope, allowing your eyes to move from one word to the next.)

ATP is generated by the cell in two pathways: fermentation (glycolysis) or respiration (aerobic mitochondrial energy generation with oxygen). Glycolysis starts with one molecule of glucose, and through a series of ten steps, transforms it into two molecules of pyruvate. Once pyruvate is generated, the cell has a decision to make. It can take pyruvate and shuttle it into the mitochondria, where it will begin the respiratory energy cycle – the highly efficient process that employs oxygen to generate a staggering twenty-three molecules of ATP. Alternately, the cell can ferment pyruvate, an inefficient method of energy production that produces only two molecules of ATP and generates a waste product, lactic acid. A healthy cell could convert pyruvate to lactic acid for a good reason; a cancer cell could do the same for a bad one.

To illustrate why a healthy cell might ferment sugar, consider a scenario. Say you were hiking in the wilderness, and you encountered a bear. Without thinking, you took off running as fast as you could. Your muscles demanded prodigious quantities of ATP, depleting the energetic currency quickly. As you ran, you began breathing rapidly, saturating the cells with oxygen, driving ATP production through aerobic respiration in the mitochondria to maximum capacity. But your extraordinarily high energy demands required more than the mitochondria could give through aerobic respiration alone. Although extremely efficient, the aerobic machinery is unable to adjust rapidly and generate ATP in a quick, short burst. Your mitochondria were using as much pyruvate as they possibly could, so to generate more ATP, your cells were forced to convert the excess pyruvate into lactic acid allowing sugar to continue the rapid but more inefficient pathway of fermentation. The valves opened as wide as possible, and a waterfall of glucose entered the fermentation pathway, generating a quick burst of ATP. But it came at a price. Your legs began to burn as the lactic acid built within the muscle cells. You made it to your car just in time, having spent all of your energetic reserves. As you calmed down, the valves that regulate the flow of glucose through the fermentation pathway returned to a position that allowed a steady state of glucose to enter the system, producing no more lactic acid, and just enough pyruvate to enter the respiratory cycle to meet the needs of the cell. Your cells are remarkable self-regulating chemical engines that constantly adjust for maximum economy.

As Bustamante and Pedersen discovered, rather than retaining a healthy cell's exquisite ability to regulate the amount of glucose entering the fermentation pathway, the valves of the cancer cell that regulated the flow were stuck open. The protein that catalyzed the first step of glycolysis (converting glucose into glucose-6-phosphate by tagging it with a phosphate group) is called hexokinase, and it alone determined the *how* of the Warburg effect. The *how* is the result of molecular square dance. The behavior of the cancer cell is drastically altered as one form of hexokinase "do-se-doed" into a slightly different form of hexokinase, dramatically altering the way the cell behaved. The "cancerous" version of hexokinase is a vestige of the past, the result of the evolutionary process as it moved through time. To understand where it came from or how it came into existence, we have to briefly explore the dynamics of DNA as it moved through time and space.

Evolution came up with a fascinating method to fine-tune metabolism. The body needed new material to work with, and like all things Darwinian, it started with an accident. Where there was one hexokinase gene before, suddenly, through a random process called duplication, a person was born with two copies. Essentially, nature laid out a fresh canvas for evolution to act on. Over time, as the new copy was inherited from generation to generation, mutations (variations in the nucleotide sequence) accumulated until a mutation resulted in a protein with a slightly altered function that helped the cell. This was Darwin's process of natural selection in a nutshell, the testing of new code in a given environment.

The new gene, a slightly altered copy of an existing gene but with new functionality, is called an isozyme. Isozymes are like tires. They all serve the same function but have differences that make them better under certain conditions (such as snow tires versus street tires or mud tires). Within our DNA, hexokinase exists as four different isozymes. Each catalyzes the first step of fermentation, but each is specialized for a given purpose within a given cell.

When Pedersen and a postdoctoral fellow, Richard Nakashima, peered inside the cancer cell, they noticed a drastic alteration in the way hexokinase was normally expressed. First, the cancer cell switched from its normal isoform of hexokinase to a rare form called hexokinase II. Second, the cells were producing vastly more of it. This singular molecular detail, he reasoned, could be the *how* behind the Warburg effect. Normal hexokinase is self-regulating (just as the way a full stomach sent an "I'm full" signal to the brain). As the product of the hexokinase reaction, glucose-6-phosphate, built up, it signals hexokinase to slow down; this is called product inhibition. The irreverent form of hexokinase, hexokinase II, ignores the signal to slow down and keeps the valve wide open, shoving as much glucose as it can down the fermentation pathway. In addition to the embezzlement of the body's energetic reserves, Pedersen envisions another consequence from hexokinase II's proclivity to force glucose down the cell's throat. "Lactic acid may build up, damaging surrounding normal tissue, helping pave the way for invasion and metastasis."

The normal regulatory mechanisms of the cell, as Pedersen and his students discovered, was subverted in the cancer cell, producing massive quantities of a perverted enzyme and slamming the fermentation pathway's "gas pedal" to the floor. Why would evolutionary pressures select for such a malevolent form of a normal enzyme? Hexokinase II must have provided the cell some sort of advantage in our evolutionary past. It could be as simple as allowing the prebiotic cell to survive periodic episodes of hypoxia, when a cell found itself in an environment with little oxygen. It was a "nursemaid" version of an enzyme, there to pull the cell through the difficult moments that undoubtedly occurred across our tenure on the planet. Today, hexokinase II might be the enzymatic version of the appendix—a body part that served a function at one time, but no longer does. As the outdated remnant was dragged through time, it transformed into something else, something malicious. The evolutionary process that created the component had yet to slough it off, leaving it hanging in the wind, allowing it to fester and decay.

Even if the cancer research community at large, with its myopic focus on DNA, ignored Pedersen and his students' discovery of hexokinase II, somebody was paying attention. A serendipitous melding of Pedersen's discovery with an emerging technology led to one of the most important breakthroughs in cancer diagnostics, one that has likely helped save untold numbers of lives.

PET Scan

In the 1970s, the nascent technology of positron-emission tomography (PET) scanning was floundering. The problem was not with the detectors, the problem was finding something worth detecting. Those seeking utility for the device needed a compound that not only the detector could see but one that concentrated itself at the site of diseased tissue, allowing for contrast between normal tissue and diseased tissue. The answer came from Pedersen's lab's discovery of the cancer cell's conversion to and overexpression of hexokinase II.

Once hexokinase II "tagged" glucose with a phosphate molecule, it was trapped inside the cancer cell. The hyperactivity and overexpression of hexokinase II resulted in cancer cells that were bloated with glucose. Here was the contrast between normal and diseased tissue needed for the diagnostic application of a PET scan. All that was then needed was a form of labeled glucose that the detectors could pick up, and it came shortly in the form of fluorodeoxyglucose (FDG), a molecule that looked like glucose but had a single oxygen atom replaced by an isotope of fluorine. This was an atom that would provide a signal.

Pedersen recalled a link between his discovery of hexokinase II and the development of PET scanning. "In the late 1970s, I was invited to give a seminar on hexokinase II at the NIH. And this man named Giovanni Di Chiro was in the audience, he was in a wheelchair, and he was very interested in what I was talking about—and then the use of FDG to detect cancer in PET scans came shortly after. I can't draw a direct line between my discovery of hexokinase II and the PET scan, but one way or the other the discovery of hexokinase II led to it." PET scanning revolutionized cancer diagnostics. To this day, no imaging technology is able to differentiate living, actively metabolizing cancer with the accuracy of the PET scan. "CT scans can image a spot, but they can't tell you if the cancer is alive or dead. PET scans are the only way to detect actively metabolizing tumors," Pedersen said.

Soon after its development, the technology made its way into virtually every cancer center across the globe, allowing for the diagnosis and tracking of untold numbers of cancer patients.

After fasting for six hours, a patient undergoing a PET scan is injected with FDG and told to lie still so that the glucose-like compound isn't taken up by muscle, creating artifacts that confuse the image. For an hour, the patient lies quietly while the glucose-analog diffuses through the body. Because of hexokinase II, the labeled glucose begins to concentrate inside cancer cells. After an hour has passed, when the patient is exposed to the detector, an elegant cascade of subatomic reactions occurs. A positron emitted from the fluorine atom collides with a nearby electron, annihilating both, but in the process, emitting a gamma ray that is converted to a photon (light). The detector then casts forth bright spots that illuminate the source: the tumor.

The process of a PET scan was a dramatic visualization of cancer's grotesquely voracious appetite for glucose. The scan was evidence of cancer's perverted metabolism, the Warburg effect, and Pedersen's unruly enzyme hexokinase II. Oncologists all over the globe read millions of PET scans, staring at the quality that Warburg and Pedersen had claimed defined cancer. Ironically, Pedersen, the star researcher who was largely ignored, inadvertently, together with his students, provided the cancer community with a tangible, visual target that could be exploited. They had been staring at it every day.

A New Era

Meanwhile, as Pedersen carried Warburg's baton, the first realization of the promised targeted drugs was about to come to fruition. It was the first step away from the indiscriminate first generation of chemotherapy and toward a modern, rational era that promised to be more effective and less toxic.

In contrast to the wall of silence that greeted Pedersen's work, the first targeted drug, Herceptin, was carried to term in a charged environment of worldwide anticipation. Herceptin carried the weight of Atlas. It was saddled with soaring expectation—it was a drug of the future, the first product of purely rational drug design. The path from idea to FDA approval contained all the drama and vicissitudes of a Hollywood production: heroes, villains, rich philanthropists, impassioned activists, desperate cancer patients, and stoic visionaries. In the end the story was told in television shows, newspapers, and books, and it was even made into a movie.

With the discovery that cancer originated by mutations to proto-oncogenes, the map to targeted drugs was established. Critical "driver" oncogenes had to be identified. That was the easy step. Figuring out the structure and function of the oncogenes' protein products would be more difficult, and the next step, designing drugs to target the dysfunctional proteins, would be even harder yet. But the inherent logic of the process was laid out, despite the obstacles it might contain. The path to drugs was clear. Scientists knew what they had to do.

During the 1980s, Weinberg was perhaps the scientist most efficient at identifying oncogenes. He was so good at finding oncogenes that he had achieved no small measure of fame (one author described the fame Weinberg achieved, "in the *People* magazine definition of the word"). Though he had yet to win a Nobel Prize, he was "as lavishly decorated as the joint chiefs of staff." His combination of popular and vocational fame meant that he was the "guy industry turned to when they felt flush and philanthropic."

In 1982, Weinberg's laboratory discovered another oncogene that was isolated from rats bearing a tumor called a neuroblastoma—the lab called the oncogene "neu." Neu had a quality that distinguished it from other oncogenes: it possessed traits that made it the perfect target for rational, targeted drug design. Most of the oncogene products discovered in Weinberg's lab coded for proteins that were isolated to the cytoplasm of the cell, the vitreous fluid filling the interior of the cell. With most of the oncogenic targets comfortably protected in the cell, the scope of possible drug candidates was compressed to those able to breach the cell's membrane barrier before seeking out the target—not a trivial task. But neu was different. The gene neu transcribed a protein that was designated to become a receptor on the outside of the cell. The receptor received a signal when a specific growth factor docked onto it, the receptor then relayed the signal to the nucleus, telling the cell to divide. From a drug design perspective, neu's accessibility was key. It was low-hanging fruit, positioned so that drugs had easy access to it.

Months after the discovery of neu, Weinberg published his finding, but incredibly, neu's potential as a drug target was left out. Somehow, its therapeutic potential escaped Weinberg and the others in his lab. With so many new oncogenes being discovered and so many pieces to connect, his attention was miles away in the theoretical clouds of cutting-edge cancer theory. "We just missed it," Weinberg said when speaking of neu's potential as a drugable target. For the time being, its potential was left hanging. But not for long.

Soon the human version of neu was discovered in an entirely different context: under the ceiling of a profit-driven pharmaceutical company. This time the utilitarian nature of neu was not missed, because it was the impetus behind the search in the first place. The human version of neu resembled another known gene, the epithelial growth factor receptor. This was an antenna-like molecule sitting on the surface of the cell that, like neu, when stimulated by its hormonal counterpart, sent a signal to the nucleus to divide. The new oncogene was called human epithelial receptor (Her-2). (It is now referred to as Her-2/neu, acknowledging its codiscovery.) The context of its rediscovery, from the theoretical ambiance of an academic lab to that of a goal-oriented company that had to answer to shareholders, drastically altered its trajectory.

By the late 1970s, the revolution in molecular biology had spun out a new breed of pharmaceutical company dedicated to capitalizing on the promise of targeted cancer therapy. It was a stark departure from the typical pharmaceutical companies that sold everything from Band-Aids to baby food. A new generation of companies with laser-like focus began to pop up on the coasts next to cutting-edge universities.

South San Francisco's Genentech was one such company. Drawing from the innovative culture of the Bay Area, talent moved seamlessly from the halls of the university to the halls of Genentech. Even Genentech's conception was unique. The company didn't start with the discovery of a drug. It started with a process, or a technology to make drugs and an infusion of venture capital. The name, Genentech, was derived from Genetic Engineering Technology, an exciting technology discovered in the late 1970s, used to "cut and paste" almost any gene into the genome of bacteria cells, thereby transforming them into factories capable of churning out prodigious amounts of the desired protein. Before Genentech, drugs like insulin were obtained by the clumsy and inefficient process of extraction from cow and pig guts. It was so inefficient that it took eight thousand pounds of ground pancreases to extract a single pound of insulin. After Genentech, the human insulin gene was spliced into bacterial cells, subverting them into remarkably efficient insulin-producing machines—a much cleaner and streamlined manufacturing method.

A decade after its inception, Genentech found itself in an uncomfortable position. It had revolutionized the process of manufacturing protein drugs, but after ten years of dazzling growth, drugs to manufacture ran out. The company had three blockbusters to its name: insulin for diabetics, a clotting factor for hemophilia, and growth hormone for a variety of childhood growth problems. Genentech was fantastic at one aspect of pharmaceutical development, but it was not in the tricky, high-risk, high-reward business of developing new drugs – at least not until the company ran out of proteins to manufacture. To design a new drug, first a target was needed, something Genentech was not accustomed to searching for. To stay relevant, the company had to shift focus. Again tapping the innovative talent in the Bay Area, the company launched a department dedicated to discovering drug targets.

German-born Axel Ullrich, a passionate scientist with a rugged charm enhanced by a German accent, was assigned to find drug targets. He was trained as a postdoc at the University of San Francisco, and the supercharged atmosphere that enveloped the Bay Area in the late seventies and eighties infected him. Varmus and Bishop were just down the hall. Ullrich's transition from academia to pharmaceutical company particularly suited his can-do nature and the culture at Genetech made the move easy. Genentech retained the free-flowing, uninhibited atmosphere of academia, scientists were largely given free reign.

When Ullrich began his search for oncogenes to target, he had a head start. He had already isolated and cloned a mutated form of a growth receptor thought to be responsible for causing blood cancer in chickens. In the world of molecular cancer biology, this was a breakthrough. For the first time, a connection between a mutated growth receptor and cancer was made, linking cause to effect. Using this example Ullrich began to look for a growth receptor responsible for cancer in humans. His search paid off when he teased out Her-2, the homolog of Weinberg's oncogene neu. Unlike Weinberg, Ullrich recognized the potential of his discovery. It was a clear oncogene *and* it was a sitting-duck, the long-imagined fantasy of rational drug design.

Ullrich had his target, but he had more obstacles to overcome. He would have to see what types of cancer Her-2 was active in, and then he would have to design a drug that blocked the Her-2 receptor. The process from target to drug was propelled by a series of fortuitous events. Puzzled by the first problem—how to determine which cancers were driven by Her-2—an answer came from a chance meeting in the Denver Airport.

Ullrich was on his way home after presenting a seminar on Her-2 at the University of California Los Angeles (UCLA). Dennis Slamon, an oncologist with a PhD in cell biology and a self-reported "murderous" obsession for curing cancer, was also at the airport, waiting for his plane. Slamon had just attended Ullrich's lecture in LA, and as he waited, he mulled over a solution to Ullrich's problem of which cancers Her-2 was active in. The scientists struck up a conversation. Ullrich had the oncogene, but he didn't have the tissue samples to test it with. Slamon did. His compulsion to cure cancer included a healthy obsession.

He collected samples of tumors of all kinds, saved in a freezer, for no other reason than he felt they might prove useful someday.

Over drinks, they plotted their course. Ullrich would send Slamon DNA probes for Her-2. Slamon would then test his samples to determine which ones, if any, expressed the product of the oncogene, answering the question of which cancers were driven by Her-2. Ullrich described the events that led to Herceptin as "an amazing amount of luck."

Once home, Slamon got to work. After exhaustively probing his samples, he called Ullrich. "We've got a hit," he said. Ullrich's probe had found its target, Her-2, in some of Slamon's breast and ovarian cancer samples. The next step was to determine what Her-2 was doing in the samples, *how* it was causing cancer. Typically, oncogenes were mutated versions of normal genes, resulting in defective protein products, but Her-2 operated by a different mechanism. It amplified itself by duplicating itself over and over again, like a copy machine with its "copy" button stuck. It transformed normal cells into cancerous ones by "overexpression." A normal breast cell might contain fifty thousand Her-2 receptors on the surface of the cell. The breast cancer cells that "lit up" Ullrich's probe contained up to 1.5 million receptors.

Her-2 wasn't mildly overexpressed on the cancer cells, it was grotesquely overexpressed. The result was cells that were hideously hypersensitive to the presence of growth factors—cells primed to misinterpret a normal signal to divide. But not all Slamon's breast and ovarian samples contained the amplified Her-2 gene. Only about one in five did, and this allowed him to categorize breast cancer into two camps: Her-2 positive and Her-2 negative. All the evidence pointed to Her-2 being a legitimate transforming oncogene, but with the stakes so high—it took more than $100 million to bring a drug to market—the research pair had to be sure.

Mutations within the DNA of cancer cells could be divided into two groups: drivers and passengers. Alterations of designated drivers did what the name suggested: they drove cancer. Passengers, on the other hand, didn't transform a cell but were only along for the ride. Ullrich and Slamon had to make sure that Her-2 was a driver and not a passenger. Slamon was in the position to make the determination, by observing whether there was a difference clinically between Her-2 positive and Her-2 negative cases of breast cancer. Carefully following patients in both camps revealed something remarkable: Her-2 positive cases resulted in a more aggressive and virulent form of cancer with a worse prognosis, exactly what would be expected if Her-2 was a driver. Ullrich performed another experiment to test the capacity of Her-2 to act as a driver. He sprinkled the Her-2 gene over normal cells and manipulated them into taking up the new gene and incorporating it into their DNA. This resulted in the same overexpression observed in the breast cancer samples. Subverted by the overexpression of Her-2, the cells ignored the intricate signals of controlled cellular division and turned into crazed proliferators. Her-2 alone marched the cells down the path to malignancy. It seemed as though Ullrich and Salmon had the target Varmus and Bishop had promised. Now all they needed was a bullet.

The creative revolution occurring in molecular biology resulted in another profound breakthrough that harnessed the remarkable qualities of the immune system. The immune system is the only barrier between us and the relentless assault of the microbial world. It is a battle-hardened collaboration of specialized cells honed through millions of years of all-out war. The immune system's ability to selectively attack foreign invaders with specificity left immunologists in awe. Nature's version of "drug design" made our attempts look silly. The immune system is a sophisticated cellular militia that contains all the elements of a modern military. Cells called macrophages act like tanks. Wielding an imposing armament of weapons, they chase down enemies and unleash vicious assaults. Commander cells direct the battle, calling forth troops and orchestrating flanks, surprise attacks, and a gamut of brilliant maneuvers, honed through eons of experience. The immune system also comes equipped with targeting missiles called antibodies. They are fired from the outer membranes of specialized cells called b-cells that display an inconceivably vast armament, able to target almost every virus and bacteria on the planet. In the midst of an infectious assault an activated b-cell turns into a biological machine-gun, churning out approximately 2000 antibodies per second. It was the antibodies that caught the attention of researchers—specifically, their ability to target any conceivable invader. To researchers trying to develop drugs, they were long sought after "magic bullets."

The idea of targeted drugs captured the imagination of biologists as far back as 1908 when German scientist Paul Ehrlich popularized the concept of a "magic bullet." He imagined a compound designed to selectively target disease-causing organisms. His inspired vision of medicine became reality in the late twentieth century when rather than trying to engineer targeted drugs themselves, researchers employed the immune system to do it for them. They found that they could coax antibody-producing cells (b-cells) to do their bidding. They injected a mouse with the desired target, causing the immune system of the mouse to scale up the b-cells armed with the antibody targeted to the foreign substance. They then isolated the b-cells from the spleen of the mouse and fused them with a cancerous myeloma cell in a sort of arranged marriage. They capitalized on the cancer cell's hyperactive growth, harnessing its perversion for utility. The hybrid cells were transformed into factories that churned out prodigious amounts of an antibody that could be targeted to virtually anything. Once manufactured, isolated, and purified, the antibodies were called monoclonal antibodies. Here was the magic bullet they needed.

Ullrich requested something from the experienced immunology department at Genentech: a monoclonal antibody targeted to Her-2.

With the magic bullet soon in hand, he performed one more simple experiment. In a petri dish, he treated Her-2 positive breast cancer cells with the monoclonal antibody. The antibodies performed their singular task with exquisite precision. They honed in on the Her-2 receptor, binding to it, covering its surface like a tarp, and blocking its ability to receive any signal to grow from the outside. The antibody brought the growth of the cancer cells to a screeching halt. When Ullrich washed the antibody from the surface of the cell, the growth resumed like nothing had happened, unequivocally proving the antibody's efficacy and mechanism of action. When recalling the simplicity and powerful implications of the experiment, Slamon said, "It was fantastic."

Ullrich and Slamon had all the proof they needed, but they had the formidable task of convincing the top brass at Genentech to gamble $100 million on their idea, a task that proved to be Ullrich's undoing. Unable to convince management of the potential of their concept, Ullrich became increasingly frustrated. His disenchantment spiraled until he quit and moved to other academic and commercial pursuits.

Raised by an Appalachian coal miner, Slamon retained the stubborn, gritty determination that flowed through the veins of humble, bootstrapping families. Unlike Ullrich, Slamon dug in and was going to see the endeavor to the end no matter what. He was about to be on the receiving end of some remarkably good luck.

In 1982, Slamon was a red-faced, junior attending physician treating a man with recurring Hodgkin's disease. Like every other type of cancer, Hodgkin's carried a much worse prognosis upon reoccurrence. The patient was Brandon Tartikoff. He was thirty years old and NBC's new "golden boy of programming." Tartikoff either conceived of or championed hits like *The Cosby Show, The Golden Girls, Miami Vice, Cheers,* and *Seinfeld*, and he put NBC on top of the ratings.

Tartikoff's treatment included nine cycles of chemotherapy over the course of one year. In that time, remarkably, he transformed NBC *and* fathered a child, all in the midst of a chemotherapeutic-induced fog. The struggle caused the Tartikoffs and Slamon to grow close; even their kids became friends.

In 1986, four years after the chemo had ended and Tartikoff's two-year checkup came back clear, his wife, Lilly, wanted to do something for Slamon. She felt that Slamon had saved her husband's life, and she wanted to pay him back by donating to his research. Slamon insisted that her only obligation was to pay the bills. Every time Lilly tried to donate to Slamon's research, he refused. This went on for two years – Lilly trying to settle her perceived debt, and Slamon refusing. In 1989, Lilly wouldn't take no for an answer. "I don't like to owe anybody anything," Lilly said. "He saved Brandon's life, and this was payback." She called Slamon. "I'm sick of this no, no, no. I'm going to do something for cancer, I'm not just doing it for you."

Her persistence wore Slamon down. When he finally agreed, Lilly began a money-raising crusade. She solicited her billionaire friend Ron Perelman, the owner of Max Factor and Revlon. "You're making all this money from women, and you should give some back," she told him. Her persistence eventually convinced Perelman. He wrote a check for $2.5 million for Slamon's research. Overnight, Slamon became the best funded researcher at UCLA.

The infighting about Herceptin continued at Genentech. The biotech company was reluctant make an "all in" bet on the drug. Slamon and his Revlon money (which ended up totaling more than $13 million from 1989 to 1997) resolved the issue. It provided the push that Genentech needed to tip the risk-reward ratio in its favor. "Without Denny Slamon and his Revlon money, there would be no Herceptin," a Genentech executive said. With it, the world's first targeted drug was born.

The amalgam of a cutting-edge biotechnology firm, Hollywood money, and the promise of a targeted cancer drug proved too seductive for the press to ignore. No cancer drug had ever been greeted with such fanfare. Well-known breast cancer specialist Craig Henderson described Herceptin as "the first step in the future," away from the "poisons" of the past. The *New York Times* called it "a significant medical breakthrough" and said that Herceptin "opened a new frontier in cancer therapy." Herceptin inspired people to quote Winston Churchill. "Now this is not the end. It is not even the beginning of the end. But it is perhaps the end of the beginning," Dr. Mary-Claire King, the American Cancer Society professor of genetics wrote in the introduction of Robert Bazell's book, *HER-2: The Making of Herceptin, a Revolutionary Treatment for Breast Cancer*. The platitudes were everywhere: "a whole new era of cancer treatment," "groundbreaking," and "revolutionary."

In the spring of 1998, ASCO, the professional organization of cancer specialists, held its annual meeting at the downtown convention center in Los Angeles. Herceptin had completed its fitful journey through clinical trials. The glamorous, famous drug was ready for its unveiling. Typically the doctors shuffled from presentation to presentation, going through the motions, but on this Sunday afternoon, the vast majority, eighteen thousand strong, squeezed into an auditorium to hear Slamon give the results of Herceptin's clinical trial. It was the marquee event.

A hushed silence greeted Slamon as he made his way to the podium. He began with the tumultuous history of the drug but couldn't tell the entire story of what it took to get there, including the collective efforts of Pott, Hansemann, Rous, Varmus, and Bishop. The journey transcended generations of effort. The moment was the manifestation of the impeccable logic that guided Herceptin's engineering from target to drug.

The adjectives describing Herceptin and all the pomp and ceremony were without meaning if the drug didn't meaningfully impact breast cancer patients. Slamon paused before delivering the results. "Herceptin demonstrates a clear benefit in every conceivable index of response. Response rates compared to standard chemotherapy had increased by 150 percent. Herceptin shrunk half of the tumors in the women treated compared to a third in the control arm."

Viewed from a different angle, Slamon's words sounded different. Albeit a convenient way to make a drug sound better than it may be, tumor shrinkage is meaningless to those fighting for their lives. It was a sanitized method of measuring a response, a statistic scrubbed clean of anything meaningful. To say "150 percent" when describing the results of a drug sounded good, but the only issue that mattered was survival. It was not clear whether Slamon gave the unsanitized version of Herceptin's results at the conference. If he did, it would have gone like this: "Herceptin is able to extend the life of a metastatic breast cancer patient by four months." A decade later, a follow-up study revealed that adding Herceptin to standard chemotherapy was able to increase absolute differences in overall survival by 2.9 percent at four years, 5.5 percent at six years, 7.8 percent at eight years, and 8.8 percent at ten years. This was significant to the fraction of patients who fell into the percentage saved but maybe not worthy of the hyperbole showered on the drug.

Mark Twain said, "Facts are stubborn, but statistics are more pliable." Beyond the statistical sledgehammer—that the most-anticipated drug provided a marginal benefit in overall survival in maybe 15 to 20 percent of breast cancer cases—was an unspoken observation.

In Ullrich's experiment, adding the Her-2 gene to normal cells turned them into cancer cells, establishing the fact that Her-2 alone could cause cancer. Other labs offered further proof that Her-2 could make a normal cell cancerous. Philip Leder at Harvard Medical School bred a strain of mice that overexpressed Her-2 from birth. The mice developed breast cancer at an unusually high rate. The tumors dissolved when treated with the antibody. Mike Shepard (who took over the Her-2/neu program when Ullrich resigned) described the process succinctly: the program was a blueprint for the proper biotech method. "First you understand the molecular events that give rise to a dangerous cancer. Then you look at that pathway, and based on technology that you have in your hands right now, you design in your head a treatment," Shepard said. The overexpression of the Her-2 gene was the molecular event determined to cause or "drive" a certain subset of breast cancer. Herceptin smothered it and choked it off, neutralizing the event determined to be the cause, yet it was of marginal benefit. Something was clearly wrong.

If Herceptin was not a cure, or not translating into substantial benefit in life extension, something else was driving the cancer. The impeccable logic that guided the creation of Herceptin contained a fatal flaw. If the overexpression of Her-2 was the singular cause of a subset of cancer and Herceptin was the antidote, by extension, the women should be cured.

Nobody was talking about that after the ASCO meeting concluded and Herceptin's unveiling was over. All those involved in creating Herceptin were there to celebrate. The drinks flowed freely. They *did* have a lot to celebrate, because the exhausting journey for the FDA approval of Herceptin was complete. Over the next ten years, the drug put almost $6.7 billion into Genentech's coffers.

An Old Target Is New Again

During the late 1990s, as Herceptin dominated the headlines of oncology, behind the scenes, Pedersen was methodically elucidating cancer's perverted metabolism. As far back as 1978, he had established that relative to normal cells, tumor cells had fewer mitochondria, and the ones he did find were terribly distorted, proving that tumor cells had a reduced capacity to produce energy aerobically. In 1977, his laboratory isolated the metabolic defect responsible for the Warburg effect: the hijacking of normal hexokinase by hexokinase II, followed by its monstrous overproduction. In 1986, his group and another group at the University of Maryland, headed by Marco Colombini, noticed that they were doing similar research and decided to collaborate. Together they showed that hexokinase II didn't exist in isolation; it bound to another mitochondrial-bound protein called the voltage dependent anion channel (VDAC). VDAC acts as a gateway for molecules (like ATP) to enter and leave mitochondria. Additionally, VDAC serves a functional role in the process known as apoptosis, "programmed cell death," allowing the release of a trigger molecule, cytochrome c, which initiates a cascade of events that culminate in the death of the cell.

A variety of cellular insults trigger a cell to undergo apoptosis. It is a highly refined and organized process designed to remove damaged cells quickly and efficiently, maintaining the fidelity of the organism and preventing the buildup of excessive waste, which could result in disease. Apoptosis is a critical cellular process, the importance of which is often underappreciated, but it also requires an organism to strike a precarious balance. The balance between cell growth and cell death is a tightrope the body must walk everyday with billions of cells condemned to death through apoptosis and billions of cells dividing to replace them. If the tenuous relationship shifts too far toward cell death, degenerative conditions like Parkinson's disease, Alzheimer's disease, and Amyotrophic lateral sclerosis (ALS) can occur. If shifted too far toward growth, cancer may occur.

The laboratories of Pedersen and Colombini discovered that hexokinase II was binding with VDAC. When bound to Hexokinase II VDAC locked the gate, preventing the release of cytochrome c therby preventing apoptosis and effectively immortalizing the cell – one of the most salient and awe-inspiring qualities of the cancer cell. However, unlike the overexpression of the oncogene Her-2/neu, which occurred in only a fraction of cases of breast cancer, the overexpression of hexokinase II occurred in virtually every cancer cell. In one fell swoop, the switch from normal hexokinase to hexokinase II not only allowed cancer cells to compensate for the energy lost due to loss of and damage to mitochondria, but it also immortalized the cancer cell, turning it into a voracious, gritty, enduring, version of a normal cell.

Pedersen's lab then made another discovery in 2003. In addition to its hysterical consumption of glucose and its impediment of apoptosis, hexokinase II positioned itself perpendicular to a protein called ATP Synthasome, a rotating machine-like protein that belched out the cellular energy currency, ATP. Hexokinase II's positioning allowed it to steal ATP before it had the chance to escape, putting the cancer cell's insatiable appetite for glucose before other cellular needs. Like a plundering pirate, hexokinase II steered its ship next to and then tethered itself to the side of a merchant ship rife with treasure, unabashedly stealing its booty.

Throughout the 1970s, 1980s, and 1990s, and into the new millennium, while the genetics of cancer took center stage, Pedersen continued to uncover the details of the Warburg effect. For a disease that was thought to be a tornado of genetic chaos, his image of cancer was one of organization and coordination. It wasn't incomprehensible, it was precise and simple. A single molecular transition to a parasitic isozyme was largely responsible for two hallmark features of cancer: the Warburg effect and evasion of apoptosis. And unlike Her-2, it wasn't in a fraction of a single cancer type (one of two hundred different types, each one its own distinct disease). It was in all of them, just as the PET scans showed.

The potential of hexokinase II as a therapeutic target was not lost on Pedersen. And as the millennium approached, he decided it was time to zero in on it. He shifted the focus of his lab from basic cancer research to developing therapies using what they had learned, from basic science to applied science. But as seductive as the target was, it was surrounded by a moat. Even if Her-2/neu was a fleeting and impotent target, the important quality that it possessed, from a drug-design perspective, was accessibility. It hung in plain sight on the outer surface of the cell.

Pedersen faced a far greater challenge in attacking hexokinase II directly, because it sat comfortably protected inside the cell. To try to get to it, rather than target it directly, he attempted a backdoor approach, targeting hexokinase II from the level of gene expression. If he could prevent the gene from being transcribed into its protein product, he reasoned, maybe he could prevent its gross overexpression. This would turn off the Warburg effect *and* reestablish a path for the damaged cell to kill itself through apoptosis.

To do this, he employed a technique called antisense RNA. Theoretically, a single strand of RNA, complementary to the single-strand of hexokinase II messenger RNA, would bind—similar to Varmus and Bishop's molecular "fishing pole"—and physically obstruct its translation into protein. It was a technique designed to "shoot the messenger" and prevent the final protein from being manufactured. But, like many others, Pedersen discovered that the technique was difficult to implement. As one commentator put it, "Antisense RNA is a technique gorgeous in concept but exasperating in use."

As Pedersen floundered trying to get the technique to work, a new postdoc came to work in his lab in 1991. The lively South Korean, Young Hee Ko, would completely change his life.

Ko entered his lab with glowing recommendations. Four of her former professors wrote Pedersen on her behalf, and her doctoral thesis advisor, Bruce McFadden, wrote that one of her research proposals was "the best and most original...[he] could remember in twenty five years at

Washington State. [Dr. Ko] is the most original doctoral student that he had in 25 years." He went on to say, "Personally, Dr. Ko is delightful. She is very modest and self-effacing yet she is developing good critical powers. She is a very considerate lab colleague." A member of Ko's thesis committee, Ralph G. Yount (a president of the American Society of Experimental Biologists), wrote, "She is personally somewhat self-effacing but intellectually aggressive. I feel she would fit into almost any lab with little trouble. She has my highest recommendation. I wish she had worked for me!" Ko's postdoctoral application came with "the highest recommendations I had ever seen," Pedersen said.

Pedersen feared that the competitive environment of Johns Hopkins might prove difficult for Ko. "My first impression from her petite stature was that other students may try to take advantage of her. However, I soon learned that she had no problem in defending her turf." Once she settled in with a project, Pedersen realized that Ko's extraordinary recommendations were perhaps understated. Her small stature veiled an unrelenting focus, vigor, and capacity to work long hours. "She has never taken a vacation; she works seven days a week. She comes in at six or seven o'clock in the morning...and goes home sometimes after midnight. If you want verification of that, you can just ask the guards," Pedersen told a reporter from *The Baltimore Sun*. "She moves passionately forward with her projects. She moves at lightning speed and works relentlessly day and night until she completes her objectives." The man who overcame any deficiencies, perceived or otherwise, through gritty work ethic alone found himself awestruck by his new postdoc's "superhuman" work ethic.

A South Korean by birth, Ko received an undergraduate degree from Kon-Kuk University in Seoul in 1981. The next year, she immigrated to the United States and enrolled in the nutritional physiology Master's program at Iowa State University, where she graduated in 1985. Yet even with a Masters degree, Ko felt unsatisfied. She had grown to feel that nutrition only skimmed the surface and craved a "deeper understanding of the way life operated" at the most fundamental level, so she enrolled in the PhD program of biochemistry at Washington State University and completed it in 1990.

When Ko entered Pedersen's lab as a postdoc, the laboratory was in the midst of several projects, one of which was researching the specific pathology of cystic fibrosis. Other labs had isolated the singular cause of cystic fibrosis: a mutated form of a protein known as cystic fibrosis transmembrane conductance regulator (CFTR). Inherited mutations in both copies of the gene left a cell unable to regulate the transport of chloride and sodium ions across membranes, a fundamental process. Victims of the inherited disease experienced a mosaic of symptoms such as lung infections, gastrointestinal problems, and endocrine issues.

Ko was assigned the task of finding out why the mutated protein was dysfunctional, a task particularly well suited to the skills she acquired while earning her PhD. True to her nature, she dove into the project with reckless abandon. Seven years and seven publications later, she and Pedersen felt that they had found the reason behind cystic fibrosis's faulty protein. "It was a localized folding problem resulting in dysfunctional CFTR," Ko said, summing up the years of research in a single sentence. The victims of cystic fibrosis had a faulty codon that resulted in a missing amino acid or the wrong amino acid within the CFTR protein, thus changing its three-dimentional arcitecture and rendering it dysfunctional.

As the new millennium approached and the work on cystic fibrosis completed, Pedersen directed Ko to his lab's marquee endeavor: cancer. To treat cancer, they knew what they had to do. They had to attack hexokinase II, the protein they felt was the beating heart of cancer. Pedersen set Ko on a task with a single focus: by whatever means possible, isolate and inhibit hexokinase II. By now it was clear to him that

Ko was special. They had been working together for a long time, and Pedersen had developed a new appreciation of her, describing her as "simply the best scientist that has ever worked in my laboratory in its thirty-four-year history." As such, he knew he was better off stepping aside—for the creative process to work, it was best to surround a goal with an empty matrix so that the imagination could approach the center unencumbered. As he expected, she attacked her goal with the vigor she was known for.

Ko recognized the futility of targeting hexokinase II with the antisense RNA method. "I suspected the antisense RNA wouldn't work," she said. Rather than emulate Pedersen's backdoor approach, she set out to find something that might inhibit hexokinase II directly. Like Pedersen, she faced the vexing problem of getting something into the cancer cell. She began working the problem backward, looking at the target before deciding on the bullet. By virtue of Pedersen's continuum of work, Ko knew, as Warburg proved more than seventy years earlier, that cancer cells overproduced lactic acid. She knew that the cell had to get rid of the corrosive waste product immediately, or it would kill the cell from the inside out, like carbon monoxide poisoning from an idling car in a shut garage. Being the survivalists they were, cancer cells overproduced a membrane-imbedded protein called a monocarboxylate transporter (MCT). The porous protein acted as a door, selectively allowing lactic acid and pyruvate (pyruvate is similar to lactic acid) to enter and leave the cell.

Ko realized that cancer cells produced many more of the "doors" than normal cells. Essentially, the door for a molecule that "looked like" lactic acid or pyruvate, typically shut on normal cells, was left wide open on cancer cells. The difference was the disparity she needed and the opening she would exploit. During quiet moments, when she thought about how to take advantage of the opening, she circled back to a molecule that she had worked with while a PhD student at

Breakthroughs and Disappointments

Washington State University called 3-bromopyruvate (3BP). It was a three-carbon molecule that shared the same chemical structure as pyruvate except for a single difference: one atom of bromine replaced a hydrogen atom. She thought it was close enough that the MCT protein wouldn't be able to tell the difference. It differed by a single atom and might be able to slip through the door unnoticed like a molecular Trojan horse. In addition, the atom that distinguished 3BP from normal pyruvate might add the reactive punch needed to mortally damage hexokinase II once inside.

Ko knew it was a long shot, but it was worth a try. The idea was elegant in its simplicity, but it seemed far *too* simple. Could cancer really have left a door wide open? Could an effective therapy come from a molecule so simple, so common, and so well known that it could be ordered from the shelf at any chemical supply house? Cancer was infinitely complex—Ko had read the textbooks. It was caused by a web of pathways so tangled and intertwined that it was going to take decades, if not millennia, to sort it out. There was no way this overly simplistic line of reasoning could work, but every time she walked through the logic, she failed to find a reason why it *wouldn't* work. So unknown to everyone in the lab, even Pedersen, she ordered a batch of 3BP from a chemical supply house.

Once the package arrived, she decided to compare 3BP with a dozen other metabolites that may or may not have anticancer properties. She added the chemicals directly to cancer cells growing in a petri dish, comparing the compounds head to head. 3BP immediately jumped out as the best candidate. "Initially I was surprised by how well it worked compared to the other compounds I was screening alongside it," Ko said. Testing its cancer-fighting prowess compared to a small list of unknown compounds was one thing; but it would also have to prove that it matched up against the chemotherapeutic heavy hitters. "I ran the first assay where I compared 3BP against

carboplatin, cyclophosphamide, doxorubicin, 5-fluorouracil, methotrexate, and paclitaxel, and I thought something was wrong. 3BP was
killing the cells so much faster," Ko said. "I just couldn't believe it, so I
ran the assays, I'm not kidding, over one hundred times."

Every time she ran the assay, she saw the same stunning result—
3BP wasn't just better at killing cancer cells than conventional chemotherapy drugs, it was vastly better. Even more shocking, it was vastly
better in every type tested: brain, colon, pancreatic, liver, lung, skin,
kidney, ovarian, prostate, and breast cancer. In every sample, 3BP
dominated the list. As any cancer researcher knew, it was best not to
get excited too quickly. Testing drugs in a petri dish was one thing,
but testing them in the complex and nuanced environment of a living
organism was a different game. Many drugs that appeared great in a
petri dish either failed to work in animals or displayed an intolerable
cadre of side effects.

Having exhausted the limited experiments she could perform
in petri dishes, Ko knew it was time to tell Pedersen about 3BP and
request to try it in animals. "It will never work," he said, when she
approached him about testing 3BP in rabbits. "It's too reactive." He
knew the inherent chemistry of molecules with similar structure
imbued them with hyperreactivity, an itchy trigger finger. As he
weighed the idea of testing 3BP in animals, his initial thought was that
it might be a fool's errand at best and maybe immoral at worst. He
thought that the jittery molecule would instantly and violently react
before it had the chance to slip inside the cancer cell, most likely killing the animal in the process.

Ko talked to her mentor at Washington State University, and he
told her the same thing. "You could waste your whole career trying to
figure out how to make it less reactive," he said.

Her persistence eventually wore Pedersen down, and he agreed.
They decided to try 3BP in a rabbit model of liver cancer (rabbits

surgically transplanted with skin cancer from a common donor into their livers). Still convinced that it was a waste of time, he watched from the sidelines. "I felt sorry for the rabbits," he said. The rabbits were injected one by one. If 3BP was going to kill the rabbit, it would probably happen soon after injection. As the tense moments passed and the rabbits continued to hop around, seemingly unfazed, they realized that 3BP might not be as toxic as Pedersen had thought.

The next morning, having barely slept, Ko went to check on the rabbits. She found them in what appeared to be perfect health. They were eating, milling around, and acting as if nothing had happened.

After several uneventful days, it was time to test the results. The rabbits were sacrificed, and an autopsy was performed to see if 3BP had had any effect on the tumors. The reactive drug had not produced any of the obvious side effects that Pedersen and others had predicted. The more substantial hurdle, determining if the drug had any meaningful impact on the tumors, remained to be overcome.

They surgically removed the tumors from the control rabbits that did not receive 3BP. As expected, the slides under the microscope displayed 100 percent active, dividing, cancer cells. The next slides contained samples from the rabbits given 3BP, and what they saw was "quite dramatic," they wrote. Every sample contained almost all dead, necrotic cells. They looked at the normal liver tissue surrounding the tumors, suspecting that the battle lines may not have been perfectly drawn and the toxicity that killed the cancer cells may have bled over into the normal tissue. The margins were clean—even the surrounding liver tissue was healthy. Everywhere they looked, it appeared that the twitchy molecule spared normal tissue—lung, kidney, brain, heart, stomach, colon, muscle, and small intestine. Every tissue examined appeared unaffected. "That's when I realized we were on to something big," Pedersen said.

As exciting as the petri dish and rabbit experiments were, the next experiment proved even more so. Pedersen and Ko decided to go from the start all the way to the finish line. They would attempt to cure rats of aggressive, advanced liver cancers, thereby restoring their normal life span. Rather than a single 3BP injection, they gave multiple injections over the course of weeks, a true test to see what the drug was capable of. The trial contained two groups: one that received 3BP and a control group that did not. As expected, the control rats quickly succumbed to the aggressive cancer, living only weeks. As the last of the fourteen control rats died, the 3BP group—all nineteen rats, even the ones with the most aggressive metastatic disease—continued to live, transcending the invisible-barrier of inevitability defined by the disease.

As the weeks passed and the animals continued their regular treatments, one PET scan after the other, incomplete by themselves, began to form a picture: the rats were being cured, *completely cured*. The weeks turned into months, and the rats appeared healthier than ever. "They were enjoying life again," Pedersen said. Every rat treated with 3BP lived a normal lifespan, and the cancer never returned. "I've been in cancer research for twenty years, and I've never seen anything like this that just melts (tumors) away," a veteran cancer researcher said.

Every potential cancer drug had to go through a series of steps to get to the ultimate destination: treating humans. The road was littered with the corpses of drugs that failed the journey. Throughout the 1990s, only 5 percent of oncological drugs that entered clinical development received approval. Worse, 60 percent of the drugs that failed did so in the middle of phase three studies, after millions of dollars had been spent. Human trials were the only way forward, because they alone determined whether a drug provided any benefit.

The Good, the Bad, and the Ugly

For 3BP, the transition to a human trial was anything but smooth. Balanced on the edge with the potential to change the course for so many desperate cancer patients, 3BP became embroiled in bitter scandal. The exalted qualities of human nature, curiosity, compassion, and logic that gave birth to 3BP had their lesser relatives derail its upbringing. As Ko put it, "This is when the bad stuff started to happen." Pedersen called the discovery of 3BP and the events that followed "the good, the bad, and the ugly."

According to a Complaint filed in the United States District Court for the District of Maryland, Ko's problems began in 2002 when she was offered a three year contract to serve as an assistant professor in Johns Hopkins' Radiology Department. According to Ko, the job came embedded with an insurmountable problem. She was not given her own independent lab space, which, as a research scientist, put her in an awkward situation. The problem was summarized in the Complaint: "It is very difficult to obtain grant money to conduct medical research (approximately one in ten to fifteen grants applied for is awarded)....It is virtually always required to have one's own laboratory space in which to conduct a project or study in order to demonstrate the principle investigators independence." Ko found herself in a strange catch-22. She could apply for grants, but because she wasn't given her own lab space, she was virtually assured not to be awarded the grant money.

The smoldering problems fully ignited in the summer of 2003, shortly after the 3BP/rat study, when Ko applied for a prestigious Susan B. Komen grant to study the effects of 3BP on breast cancer. When she received word that she had been awarded the grant Ko was ecstatic. "It was one of the happiest days of my life," said Ko. She had two reasons to be happy. First, the high profile grant would allow further investigation into 3BP's cancer fighting potential, moving the compound one step closer to clinical trials. Second, with the grant, Ko was under the impression she would finally receive her much needed laboratory space. According to the Complaint, Ko had a letter from the former Chair of the Radiology Department, Dr. Robert Gayler, promising Ko laboratory and office space if she was awarded the Komen grant and if approved by [the standing Vice Dean for Research] Dr. Chi Dang.

"But my happiness only lasted one hour," said Ko. Elated by her new grant Ko approached the new Vice Dean of Research about her promised laboratory space. After meeting with Dang, Ko heard her email box ping. It was an email from the Vice Dean Dang with five others copied in, stating that Ko's grant submission was "in fact, misleading to the Komen foundation." Stunned, Ko approached the Vice Dean to find the basis of the accusation. The confusion was isolated to a single detail. According to the Complaint Dang assumed that the grant submitted to the Komen Foundation, like the vast majority of grant applications, required that an applicant already have laboratory space— the insurmountable catch-22 Ko was captured. "But the Komen grant application had no such requirement, they didn't even ask the question about lab space," said Ko. For Ko, the accusation carried more of a sting for other reasons. Years earlier, a research meeting had been convened in which faculty members were asked to discuss what they were working on. When it was Pedersen's turn he talked about his lab's exciting work with 3BP. Pedersen explained he and Ko remained cautiously optimistic 3BP might turn out to be a legitimate anti-cancer drug. According to the Complaint, the laboratory headed by Dang then "immediately requested some 3BP for use in the laboratory." As time passed, Dang's laboratory even requested Ko and Pedersen's expertise. The Complaint states that Ko spent 80 hours on one assay alone, both conducting and writing up the research for the other laboratory. On another occasion a member of Dang's laboratory visited Pedersen's lab to seek assistance from Ko regarding hexokinase II research. To Ko and Pedersen's surprise, Dang's lab was steering their efforts toward research Pedersen's lab was already focused on. Nevertheless, according to the Complaint Ko spent over 30 hours teaching a student how to assay hexokinase, saving Dang's lab an estimated 2 to 12 months' time.

Ko was shocked that with all her donated time helping others, and the fact the Komen grant application did not request information regarding the applicant's access to laboratory space, she was not being congratulated and given the laboratory space that she felt had been promised to her. Ko clearly felt she was being subjugated to a double standard. Dismayed, she demanded the Vice Dean apologize for the email stating that her application had misled the Komen Foundation. To Ko it felt like her career and research were deliberately being sabotaged. But the situation had escalated too far—both sides had become so galvanized that a compromise couldn't be reached. On April 22 Ko was handed a letter stating that her continued faculty appointment was contingent upon her receiving a psychiatric evaluation.

"I was pissed off," said Pedersen. "Here is this person trying to cure cancer and she is being treated like this." In a moment of more thoughtful reflection Pedersen isolated the problem to one of misincentives. "It is wrong to put people doing research in charge of others doing research—scientists at this level are competitive, you're just asking for trouble. Others with control of lab space were doing research which overlapped with ours, it's the perfect set-up for a bad outcome."

Pedersen had been at Hopkins long enough to know the disciplinary process Ko was being subjected to was far from perfect. "The psychiatric evaluator is likely to work with the accuser," said Pedersen. "I knew this was not going to have a good outcome. It was the first step out the door." Ko refused the evaluation because "she did not wish to be perceived as a scientist accused of having an unsound mind and any treatment of this kind could become part of her permanent record." Knowing full well refusal of the evaluation would likely result in her termination, on June 1, 2005 she filed a 108 page complaint in the United States District Court for the District of Maryland alleging discrimination, retaliation and a number of state torts claims.

In the winter of 2005, just as tempers were beginning to calm, a reporter for *The Baltimore Sun* ran an award-winning three page article about 3BP entitled: "Young researcher stalks cancer: With little life outside the lab, a Hopkins worker studies a chemical that shuts down tumors in rats." According to Ko, the top-brass at Hopkins thought it was irresponsible and premature to be touting the promise of 3BP, and in an instant the entire situation was once again ignited, starting a renewed round of friction, again hampering Ko and Pedersen's work. The lawsuit was finally settled in 2006. The conclusion of the lawsuit upheld two patents. The first was a patent shared between Pedersen, Ko, and an M.D. named Jean-Francois Geschwind.

In the winter of 1999 Geschwind had entered Pedersen's lab as a research science student. Laboratory experience looks good on a resume, and students often ask professors if they can help in the lab to gain bench experience. Pedersen didn't know it at the time, but looking back he said letting Geschwind into his lab was "the biggest mistake of my career." Geschwind was put on the cancer therapy project, and eventually on the 3BP/rabbit study. According to Ko's Complaint his overall contribution was to guide the catheter into the hepatic artery and "push the plunger." But "naively," said Ko, Pedersen included Geschwind's name on one of the publications relating to 3BP. Pedersen also included Geschwind on the first patent application regarding 3BP's anticancer capacity, "Not realizing that there are differences between inventorship and authorship," said Ko. So even though allegedly he had little to do with the discovery and development of 3BP, Geschwind was included on the first patent application filed. The patent, shared with Johns Hopkins University, was for the intra-arterial delivery of 3BP to treat hepatic cancer in the United States. The second patent application filed in 2006 gave Ko exclusive rights to her proprietary formulation of 3BP to treat 100% of all PET positive cancer types both within the United States and abroad. And according to Ko, the formulation is everything. The formulation alone allows 3BP to achieve the necessary concentration to treat cancer. Also, the formulation prevents 3BP from reacting too early, mitigating toxicity. With the lawsuit settled, Geschwind quickly took advantage of the first patent bearing his name. He went on to found a company called PreScience Labs. The company's stated mission: "To develop powerful, effective and safe anti-cancer agents by disrupting tumor metabolism." In 2013 the company received FDA approval for the immediate enrollment of a phase 1 study using 3BP to treat metastatic liver cancer patients. According to the company's website, and a 2013 telephone conversation with the company's president, Jason Rifkin, they are still trying to procure funding for the phase 1 trial.

In the end, the damage had been done. 3BP's delicate march toward human trials had been sidelined in a multi-year lawsuit. Ko left Johns Hopkins, leaving Pedersen's laboratory with an undeniable void—a hole in the center. The once vibrant, bustling, laboratory was without its star researcher. But the real tragedy existed beyond the hushed conversations and busy lawyers; beyond the hurt feelings, anger, sanctimony, and bitterness. The real tragedy was an ephemeral abstraction—it was the untold damage that remained hidden from view. The real tragedy was best represented by Ko's empty flasks, pipettes, and other equipment that now sat idle, and began to collect dust—the real possibility that lives might have been saved by 3BP. How many? No one will ever know.

Without her work space—the environment that had been her entire life for over a decade—Ko retreated, isolated herself, and focused on her work with a singular purpose – developing an almost maternal attachment to 3BP and its potential to help people. "I haven't done anything else with my life," admits Ko, "so this is my baby." In the summer of 2008 she felt the formula was finally ready to enter a human trial. Typically, a drug will first establish if it has any efficacy by performing a "case study" on a single individual before going on to larger trials. Ko wouldn't have to go looking for a case study; in fall of 2008 one came to her. She received an e-mail from the father of a dying son, pleading for her help. The father's name was Harrie Verhoeven, and his son was Yvar. They lived in the small town of Schjindel, in the Netherlands. After exhausting every option to treat his son's cancer, a desperate search had led him to Ko. It was his son's last chance. "It was so moving," she said. "I think 3BP really was the last chance for his son."

"If I Hadn't Seen It with My Own Eyes, I Wouldn't Have Believed It"

Almost a decade after Ko stared in amazement as 3BP made a who's who list of FDA-approved chemotherapy drugs look like amateurs (and then went through the crucible of drama), the drug with so much potential got the chance to help somebody. A human trial was necessary for the maturation of the adolescent drug. It would work, it wouldn't work, or it would prove too toxic. In any case, it would be a big step in determining the drug's future.

The story began a year earlier when, out of nowhere, Yvar noticed that he was burping a lot, an annoyance more puzzling than concerning for the teenage boy. A month passed and another, and the burping continued. "Stop burping, Yvar!" his mother scolded him, thinking that it was nothing more than the insolence of a sixteen-year-old. In another few months, what had begun as an inconvenience had progressed into a terrible annoyance; he was burping constantly. His family began to think that something might be wrong. Though it appeared to be nothing more than a mild digestive issue, they made an appointment.

The doctor agreed with the family. It presented like a mild case of intestinal gas, it could be any number of things—a stomach bug, too much spicy food, or too much soda, but it was nothing to be concerned about. He prescribed stomach acid suppressors and sent them on their way. He noted that when he palpated Yvar's stomach, the boy had some mild enlargement of the liver, but the doctor told them not to worry. Along with the intestinal gas, it would most likely pass.

Yvar settled into his normal routine, hanging out with friends and practicing taekwondo. He was one of the youngest students in the Netherlands ever to receive a black belt, and trophies and ribbons from European tournaments were scattered throughout his room.

But rather than subsiding, the burping only got worse. He burped continuously, even in the middle of sentences. The medication had not worked.

August 9, 2008, began like any other day. It was a typical summer morning, and Yvar was playing Xbox online with his American friends. "I could hear him yelling and cursing at the game from the other room," his father said. "Then I heard Yvar scream in pain, so I ran into the room, and he was clutching his abdomen. He was pale and cold and covered in sweat." His family helped him to the car and rushed to the emergency room. "He was in terrible pain," his father said.

At the emergency room, the attending doctor palpated his stomach. Yvar's liver was enlarged, as was his spleen, and his temperature was high. The doctor ordered blood work for liver enzymes, a measure of liver distress.

When the results came back, Verhoeven noticed the doctor seemed panicky. The team shuttled Yvar and his family into a separate room, where the doctor explained that the boy's enzymes were fifteen times what they should be. One possible explanation was cancer, but liver cancer at the age of sixteen was almost unheard of. Whatever the culprit was, it had transcended some fragile biological barrier with frightening speed, no gradual prelude of symptoms. Something had snapped, presenting with alarming suddenness. Scans were scheduled for the next day.

In the morning, Yvar underwent a CT scan, an MRI, and a PET scan, and all came back with the same terrible image. He had hepatocellular carcinoma. His liver was consumed by it—fist-sized masses had taken over 95 percent of the organ. The images showed that it had spread with uncommon vigor, even landing on his heart. The sudden turn of events, and the horrible quickness they unfolded in, left him and his family in shock. What a few days ago was an innocent case of unexplained intestinal gas had, in a few hazy moments, turned into the delivery of a death sentence. The tumor was far past operable, so transplant was the protocol for such a dire case. But even that was not an option, the doctors explained, because Yvar's tumor had spread so aggressively he was not considered a candidate. There was some sober talk of trying chemotherapy but less for the outcome and more because they had to try something. He was too young to be sent home to die. Even so, the doctors told him and his family the brutal truth. Yvar probably had less than three months. He probably wouldn't live to see his seventeenth birthday.

A week after the diagnosis, Yvar received a call from his doctor. Finally it was good news. Nexavar, a chemotherapeutic drug approved for kidney cancer, had received orphan drug status for liver cancer. It was a stroke of good fortune in what was a hopeless situation. Finally they could feel a scrap of hope. Even though it was largely untested and Yvar would be the youngest patient ever to receive the drug, it was something. Nexavar was one of a new generation of "targeted drugs" designed to target a cancer cell's malevolent machinery with exquisite precision. It specifically targeted tyrosine kinases, a group of proteins often implicated in the pathogenesis of cancer. But tyrosine kinases also serve healthy cells, and a drug's ability to distinguish between the two overlapping proteins determined how well the drug worked and the magnitude of side effects.

Initially the drug worked. Yvar's tumors at least halted their unrelenting expansionary march. But the initial response, as is so often the case, proved to be short- lived. The drug was a single move in a chess game, and the cancer had already countered it and moved ahead. With Nexavar no longer effective, Yvar was again hopeless. His health was in free fall. The methodical subversion of what was left of his liver was releasing a steady stream of toxic shrapnel into his bloodstream, sending him in and out of consciousness. His father quit his job at a university-related institute where he worked as a plant molecular biologist to take care of Yvar full time. He searched the Internet at night, hoping to find anything that might help. He had a head start. Because of his education and training, he knew where to look.

His search lead him to Evangelos Michelakis at the University of Alberta, the man responsible for the discovery of dichloroacetate (DCA), the molecule that had received a brief spike of attention for the preclinical promise it exhibited on a variety of cancers. "But Yvar didn't qualify for DCA, I was told," Verhoeven said.

With little time, he shifted his focus to a molecule called 3-bromopyruvate. He had heard about the preclinical work, and *The Baltimore Sun* ran a punchy article highlighting the promise of the experimental drug, explaining how the molecule rid nineteen rats of advanced liver cancer. The drug operated in a different way than traditional cancer drugs, attacking the defective metabolism of the cancer cell. Further research into the drug exposed the fact it was highly reactive and could prove dangerous if not administered correctly. It was a simple, cheap molecule readily available at most chemical supply houses and wouldn't be hard to get. He thought about ordering it himself, but he knew that the formulation was key, and the reactivity of the molecule might push Yvar over the abyss. His son's life was balanced on a knife's edge, delicately sustained by the sliver of healthy liver tissue he had left.

Verhoeven contacted Young Ko of Johns Hopkins, the woman responsible for the discovery of 3BP's anticancer ability, knowing that she knew every nuance of 3BP, the right dosage, and the proper formulation. If Yvar was to get 3BP, Ko would have to help. Time was critical, because Yvar was in awful shape, and his father knew that each day could easily be his last. As he explained the situation to Ko, she was moved to tears. She couldn't help but feel deep compassion for the desperate father and his dying son. She had come as close as she could to perfecting the formulation, crucial to keep the twitchy drug from reacting too early once in the body. She felt that 3BP was ready.

She dropped everything, channeling all her time and prodigious energy toward helping Verhoeven and his son. She needed to find a doctor willing to administer the unknown drug, and this proved harder than expected. The search devoured the one thing Yvar didn't have: time. Together with her assistants she decided on a shotgun approach and sent more than five hundred e-mails to doctors throughout the United States, explaining the situation and hoping that one of them would have the courage to administer the drug. It was a long shot. One of the hardest parts of getting a new drug through trials was finding doctors willing to take the inherent risk. When she didn't hear back from any of the requests, she turned to a friend who knew a doctor in Germany who might be willing to help. European doctors had more discretion than American doctors, and they were more inclined to try experimental drugs and procedures in patients with no other options.

Ko contacted the doctor, Thomas Vogl, at the University of Frankfurt. Vogl was a world-renowned expert in a pioneering process of drug delivery called transcatheter arterial chemoembolization (TACE), which involved snaking a tube from artery to artery until it reached the vessel directly feeding the tumor. It moved the chemotherapeutic battle line from one of random diffusion throughout the body to a direct and forceful assault. More than five hundred doctors shied away from helping with the unknown drug, but Vogl stepped up, knowing that it was Yvar's last chance. But first permission to administer the experimental drug would have to pass the University of Frankfurt's ethics board, a process that would eat away another precious month. As the weeks passed and the ethics board continued its deliberative process, Yvar's condition was dire. "The doctors had no idea how he was still alive," Verhoeven said.

Vogl decided that he had to try to buy Yvar some time—he would use TACE to try to at least pause the tumor's relentless subversion. Vogl guided a catheter on an interarterial journey beginning in Yvar's groin and landing in the vessel supplying the tumors. Vogl then delivered gemcitabine and cisplatin, two highly toxic drugs shown to evoke a slight response in liver cancer but unable to increase overall survival. "It was a desperate attempt to just get Yvar to where we could get him the 3BP, he was so sick," Verhoeven said. The cytotoxic drugs may have beaten back the tumor and bought Yvar some time, but the drugs racked him with unremitting fits of nausea, further compounding his misery.

Knowing that approval was pending, Ko traveled to Germany to help administer 3BP. When she arrived, she was shocked by what she saw. "When I got there, Yvar was in horrific shape. He was skin and bones, and his arms were yellow and bruised. He couldn't eat, and he had a feeding tube. He had to sleep sitting up because the tumors were so large they stretched his abdomen when he tried to lay back, and he was throwing up so much he didn't just have a bucket next to him, he had a barrel," Ko said.

In Vogl's office, they discussed the trial, dosage, timing, and delivery. Ko couldn't help but notice the commotion going on—men were scurrying around with what appeared to be camera equipment. She learned that a documentary was being filmed on the actress, Farrah Fawcett, and her struggle with cancer. Fawcett's battle had led her to Vogl and his TACE technique. Her cancer had spread wildly, and all attempts to combat it had proved ineffectual. Moved by her story and stoic courage, Ko urged Vogl to help her and to give her 3BP. It was too late; her cancer had spread too far and they didn't have the time to jump through the hurdles.

On February 29, 2009, a year and a month after Yvar's original diagnosis, the ethics committee agreed to allow him to be treated with the experimental drug. Vogl and Ko decided the best route of delivery was via TACE. Due to 3BP's reactivity, the closer it could be delivered to the tumor, the better. Ko's patented preparation would also be key. It was a process she likened to "adding layers, like an onion, that were peeled off one by one, delivering waves of the active drug to the cancer cells." Yvar's situation was so dire that the duo decided to inject him twice the first day for a total dose of 250 ml. "I considered checking Dr. Ko into the emergency room while we were injecting Yvar with her drug. She was so utterly consumed with nervous excitement we thought she might faint," said an assisting nurse. "In the end, she composed herself enough to remain present." There was nothing to do but wait. Ko said, "I was so nervous to finally see 3BP enter a person, and you just don't know if there are going to be side effects."

Yvar received the injection at two o'clock. By three o'clock, he was still feeling okay with no immediate side effects, unlike the other cytotoxic chemotherapies that had hit like a ton of bricks, bringing on waves of nausea. At four o'clock, there was no nausea, temperature, or rash.

At five o'clock, Yvar stirred, smacked his lips, and said, "I feel hungry." He hadn't been able to eat for months. "When he said he was hungry, we all began to cry," Ko said. "It was such an emotional moment. Maybe the drug was working that fast."

A week later, Yvar received another injection of 3BP via TACE. Again, no immediate side effects were observed, and he was allowed to return home, but a mild case of light-headedness turned into confusion. "He didn't know who we were and began acting very agitated and aggressive," Verhoeven said. By the next morning, Yvar was in a coma. "I called the hospital, explaining the situation. Basically they told me that Yvar's situation was hopeless, and I needed to just let him die." Verhoeven suspected that he knew the problem. The ambulance brought Yvar to the emergency room, and again the desperate father found himself having to convince the attending physicians to treat his son. They balked, running through the diagnosis in their minds. With end-stage liver cancer, there was nothing left to do but palliative care. His desperation persuaded the doctors to order a battery of blood work, casting a wide diagnostic net to snag the culprit. They soon had their answer: ammonia. Verhoeven had suspected as much. Yvar's sky-high ammonia levels were the result of tumor lysis syndrome, a rare syndrome caused when massive quantities of cancer cells die a sudden, disorderly death, releasing their toxic payload into the blood stream. Not only was 3BP working, it was working *too well*. The side effects of the tumor lysis syndrome proved to be transient, and Yvar woke up. The doctors watched him for a while and allowed him to go home by nightfall. "Everybody breathed a huge sigh of relief," Ko said.

When the time came for the next treatment two weeks later, they were prepared. Yvar was given Hepa-Merz, a drug that removed excess ammonia and negated the toxic effects of tumor lysis syndrome. His ammonia levels began to rise, showing dramatic evidence for the efficacy of the drug, but he remained conscious and experienced only mild nausea. The next five treatments, each given about two weeks apart, went smoothly. By the summer, four months after starting treatment with 3BP, he began to regain strength. His 24-hour feeding tube was removed, and he was enjoying the foods he liked. He regularly left his wheelchair for walks. He was hanging out with his friends, playing Xbox, and cursing at the TV as he lost himself in the moment.

In September, six months after Yvar began treatment with 3BP, Ko flew to the Netherlands to celebrate his eighteenth birthday. "It was absolutely wonderful," Ko said. "The doctors told him he wouldn't make his seventeenth birthday, and here we were celebrating his eighteenth, and he was getting stronger every day." After his ninth treatment with 3BP, Yvar went in for CT scans. The scans were compared to the images at the time of diagnosis to determine how effective the 3BP treatment had been, and the difference was stunning. The "before" images depicted a liver full of active malignancy, with the surrounding lymph nodes and spleen subverted by the disease. The "after" scans showed necrotic, encapsulated tumors surrounded by normal lymph nodes and a normal spleen. The fluid surrounding the liver, once full of free-floating malignant cells, contained none, suggesting complete eradication. There were no signs of active cancer cells, only a scorched battlefield. Even the battlefield was beginning to clear; Vogl detected evidence of liver regeneration—life emerging out of the ashes. "This is something we have never seen before," Vogl said of Yvar's regenerating liver. Every test led to the same inescapable conclusion: 3BP had eradicated Yvar's cancer.

Two months later, Yvar accepted an invitation from Pedersen and Ko to come to Johns Hopkins and speak about his experience with 3BP in front of the university's first-year medical students. He was feeling better every day, so his family planned a vacation around the event. After the talk, they would fly to Utah, rent an RV, and tour the Western United States. "We are planning on going to the Grand Canyon, which my mom wants to see. I want to go to Vegas," Yvar said to the laughing medical students as they chatted after the presentation. After the RV tour, they planned to return to Salt Lake City, where they would spend Thanksgiving with family. They would fly to New York City for another round of sightseeing before returning to the Netherlands.

The students graciously thanked Yvar and his family for coming. It was a something far outside the normal routine. "Thank you too, I've already had so much fun," Yvar said with a big smile.

Shortly after they returned home, Yvar came down with pneumonia. No one can be sure where, or how, he acquired it. He had won his war against cancer, but the fight had been costly, unfortunately nobody knew just how costly it had been—not his father, not his doctors, not Dr. Ko. So much of his liver had been subverted by the disease that even with the cancer eradicated he was left with a tiny portion of functioning liver, roughly just five percent. And although his liver was in the process of regenerating, Yvar's health was left hanging by a tenuous thread.

As Ko recited Yvar's story, she stopped numerous times, her eyes welling with tears, her voice trailing off as if imagined scenarios coursed through her mind. "If only we had kept him in a bubble until he was stronger and his liver was more mature." The antibiotics he had no choice but to take required a healthy liver to process, and they were too much for the portion of liver he had left.

Yvar did not die of cancer. A CT scan performed shortly after he contracted pneumonia told the story. There was not a living cancer cell found anywhere in his body. He was lost to the damage the cancer had done, but the distinction was meaningful. The experimental molecule that operated in an entirely different way from all other cancer drugs had done something miraculous. "If I hadn't seen these results on my own equipment, with my own eyes," Vogl said, "I would not have believed them."

In the summer of 2009, with Yvar's trial nearing its completion and four years after *The Baltimore Sun* article, word about the blockbuster potential of 3BP found its way to the top. Pedersen and Ko felt that 3BP was more than ready to enter large-scale trials and once and for all prove its efficacy to the world. Ko shared a mutual friend with billionaire David Koch. Aware of her work with 3BP, the friend informally told Koch of the excitement surrounding the new drug. During the conversation Koch expressed an interest, wondering if the drug could possibly treat prostate cancer. The mutual friend then approached Ko, relaying that Koch might be interested in funding research for 3BP's effect on prostate cancer. To move forward, Koch requested preliminary data to see if the experimental drug warranted his support. Excited by the possibility of funding, Ko got to work, quickly compiled evidence substantiating that at least within a petri dish, 3BP was active against prostate cancer.

She learned that Koch used James Watson as his science advisor, so all the data would have to flow through him. "I handed the data over to Watson and then waited to hear back," she said. The call soon came from Watson, inviting Pedersen and Ko to come to Manhattan and discuss the next step over lunch. On an unusually hot day in August, Pedersen and Ko made the three and a half hour trip to downtown Manhattan and met Watson at L'Absinthe, an expensive French restaurant on East Sixty-Seventh Street.

Ko asked Watson if he had made the recommendation to Koch to fund her research. According to Ko, Watson admitted that he hadn't said anything to Koch but had instead given the data to Lewis Cantley, Director of the Cancer Center at Weill Cornell Medical College and New York-Presbyterian Hospital (he cofounded the biotechnology company Agios, a start-up focused on the metabolism of cancer). To Ko it appeared as if Watson had handed the data to her competitor without her permission.

She was astonished. "I gave him the data in confidence," she said. "He wasn't sorry or regretful." "The lunch meeting quickly became tense," Pedersen said. "I was just trying to keep things civil."

Ko said Watson then shifted direction and offered a new proposal. He was the chairman of the scientific committee for the Champalimaud Foundation, an extremely well-funded foundation dedicated to health related research. It was founded by the late Portuguese entrepreneur Antonia de Sommer Champalimaud. "Watson proposed that Pete and I hand over the data and let the foundation 'take it from here.' He wanted to take 3BP and just have Pete and I quietly go away," Ko said. "Of course, I was reluctant."

With lunch coming to an end Watson surprised them by inviting Pedersen to come to Cold Spring Harbor in New York, the nonprofit research institute where Watson spent most of his career as the director and president, to give a seminar on 3BP. Pedersen accepted.

When the day arrived to travel to Cold Spring Harbor, Pedersen asked Ko to accompany him to help field questions. "The presentation at Cold Spring was a disaster," she said. "My computer stopped working. I've never had it stop like that. I couldn't do anything for forty-five minutes. When we finally got it working, it was in read-only mode, so all the slides were in terrible resolution—you could barely read them." In retrospect, she had a different take. "Maybe it was divine intervention, a message telling me not to reveal too much data." "After the seminar, Watson kept hovering around her, trying to get her to reveal the formula," Pedersen said. Suspicious of Watson's intentions, she kept her information closely guarded. 3BP, the molecule with high and now widespread expectations, was still unfunded.

After leaving Johns Hopkins, Ko is now at the University of Maryland BioPark. Her academic career has morphed into a fledgling biotech/pharmaceutical company called KoDiscovery LLC, exclusively focused on bringing 3BP to market. And the energetic BioPark was the perfect atmosphere for the transition. Pedersen and Ko certainly had to navigate choppy waters to get here. Some scars were obvious. Some remained hidden. One thing that survived the tumult was their working relationship. It was fatefully synergistic from the beginning. Pedersen, the last surviving member of Warburg's fraternity, mapped out the target, allowing Ko to make the connection between 3BP and the altered metabolic landscape of the cancer cell. Pedersen was the wise old mentor, Ko his star pupil. They never questioned or doubted each other. They had each other's back no matter what. But as remarkably productive as their union has been it has been equally tumultuous. The path for 3BP has been anything but smooth. Ko hasn't exactly gone looking for trouble, but she has certainly bumped into her fair share. Without question the problems encountered at Hopkins have changed her, made her more guarded and suspicious of people's intentions. "Young would do anything for the people she loves, she would walk to China for you if you asked her to," said a close friend, "But I just wish she would look forward more than backward. She needs to move on from the past."

Most of their regret came from the fact that 3BP had been unnecessarily held up by the lawsuit. A drug with vast potential sat on the sidelines for almost a decade while tremendous numbers of people suffered and died. As was the case with all fledgling drugs, funding was the biggest hurdle, and today, it is more difficult than ever. Even Pedersen had difficulty getting funding for cancer research, and two of his recent NIH applications were literally thrown in the trash without a formal review. In January 2013, at his wit's end, he sent a letter to President Obama, explaining the situation and urging him to fund clinical trials for 3BP. Not surprisingly, in the bureaucratic cobweb that exists, Pedersen received a standard "receipt" letter a year later from a staff member. The problems they had encountered after their discovery of 3BP now seemingly behind them, one has to believe that it is only a matter of time for 3BP to get the funding needed for trials.

As the day I spent interviewing Ko and Pedersen turned to night, Ko kept jumping up, scurrying through the room, occasionally leaving to take care of some detail in her laboratory. Her mind was in continuous overdrive. Rumored to work eighteen hours a day, she didn't answer when I asked her if it was true. She tilted her head to the side, neither admitting nor denying. When I received an e-mail at 2:36 a.m., it confirmed her epic work hours. "I have trouble sleeping," she said. "I can't turn off my brain." It was clear that 3BP's potential to save lives substituted for her sacrifice. When she spoke of the people she loved or helped, a warm smile took over her face. It was clear that she had developed a profound attachment to Yvar and his family and was deeply affected by his eventual death, saying, "if only we had kept him in a bubble, he would not have gotten pneumonia, and he would still be here." As deeply compassionate as she was, it was clear that she refused to be pushed around or capitulate to injustice. She would dictate her destiny without giving an inch to anyone with questionable intentions. Her desire to control her surroundings was evident everywhere—every detail of the day was planned. As the catered dinner arrived, so did some friends, a short list of confidantes in her inner circle.

The interview switched from the past to the future. Pedersen's trusted accountant and his son (also an accountant but experienced in start-up companies and the process of raising venture capital) took over the conversation about the future of 3BP. Ko had made the transition from academic scientist to CEO of her own pharmaceutical company. She rattled off FDA requirements and the process for clinical trials. To move forward with a trial involving twenty or so patients, she estimated that she needed $3 million. She had an offer, "but it was a bad one," because it grossly undervalued the potential of 3BP. But it seemed clear that it was not about the money for her. It was about recognition for her work and perhaps not wanting to give up too much control of 3BP, the drug to which she had devoted a large part of her life.

One thing stood out as amazing. Because of the nature of 3BP's target, cancer's defective metabolism, Ko could pick almost any cancer she wanted for the initial trial. "If we choose kidney cancer, because it is rare, the FDA makes it much easier, costing less for applications and taking less time," she said, "but we could also choose skin or brain." Herceptin was able to target only 20 percent of a single type of cancer, allowing it to be prescribed for approximately fifty thousand cases of cancer out of 1.7 million overall diagnoses. GLEEVEC was prescribed for fewer than nine thousand cases each year or .5 percent of all diagnoses. In theory, 3BP could target any cancer that was "PET positive" (meaning that cancer was actively fermenting glucose via over-expressed Hexokinase II). Considering that this equated to about 95 percent of all cancers (the ones that were not PET positive were probably not growing, or growing slowly), the implication was almost inconceivable. If 3BP lived up to its promise, it could be the most important discovery in humanity's battle with cancer since the dawn of time.

In the large scheme of the cancer industry, 3BP needed an almost trivial amount of money to kick things off, so why wasn't there more interest? Here was a drug that could revolutionize cancer treatments, yet where were the Ron Perelmans? Where were the patient advocacy groups that took over the front lawn at Genentech, absolutely demanding Herceptin?

Part 4

Dark Matter

"It has become axiomatic that the seeds of cancer lie in genes."
—Michael Bishop

"The important thing is not to stop questioning."
—Albert Einstein

The late nineties in the United States were defined by a meteoric euphoria over technology. It was an incandescent decade of unlimited possibility, economic expansion, and prosperity. Allen Greenspan aptly labeled it a period defined by "irrational exuberance." The tech-heavy NASDAQ shot up nearly 700 percent from 1995 to 2000, and fortunes were made overnight.

The euphoria was sparked by the nascent power of the Internet. Everyone was calling it a "new economy." Dot-com fever was pandemic. Investors convinced themselves that shell companies with no earnings, just wildly optimistic vision and a name with ".com" following it, were worth hundreds of millions in stock market valuation. The euphoria spilled over into biotechnology. Visionaries started biotech companies and attracted venture capital with nothing more than an elegantly pitched dream and a narrative of a future without disease or aging.

The cloning of "Dolly" the sheep in the mid-1990s pollinated the atmosphere. Called somatic cell nuclear transfer, the technology was Ponce de Leon's fabled fountain of youth. It was a recapitulation of ourselves in a renewed version. A biological sleight of hand was performed by extracting DNA from an adult organism's cell and transplanting it into an isolated oocyte, an egg cell, with its DNA removed. Instead of the mingling of genes that evolution used to pick and choose favorites, the embryo was a clone, an exact replica of its donor. The fertilized egg was then planted into a surrogate, where it gestated until birth. It came as a shock to most scientists that cloning was possible. The egg cell was capable of something almost magical. The egg contained unknown factors that conspired to rejuvenate the older sheep's DNA, rearranging it back to ground zero, the moment when sperm met egg, resetting the clock in a display of biological time travel—again allowing the program of life to begin its magical journey, unfolding a dazzling symphony of molecular choreography, creating a life.

The fact that DNA was so malleable, so pliable, and capable of being rejuvenated was incredible, and it opened an inconceivable spectrum of possibility. Companies sprouted up to capitalize on the unlimited possibility of the technology. Advanced Cell Technology was one company. "We are close to transferring the immortal characteristics of germ cells to our bodies and essentially eliminating aging," its founder, Michael West, told *Wired*. "That sounds spectacular, but I believe those are the facts." West wasn't alone in his belief. Calvin Harley, the head scientist at Geron, said, "We are all born young. There is a capacity to have an immortal propagation of cells the way we have evolved is to go from germ line to germ line, with our somas (bodies) the dead end carriers, but that is not inevitable."

Perhaps more than any other decade, the nineties were defined by a collective belief that we were on the cusp of a transformative new era, even though many of the dreams propagated by the visionary companies failed to materialize. Bundled in the euphoria was the belief that the explosion in biotechnology might even topple cancer.

The power of technology infected the subconscious and was on everyone's mind as President Clinton approached the podium in the East Room of the White House on June 26, 2000. He announced that the government's effort to sequence the entire human genome had completed a rough draft. Francis Collins, the head of the project, was on his left. On his right was Craig Venter, president and chief science officer of Celera Genomics, a biotech company with the loosely defined business plan of sequencing the human genome alongside the government effort.

The origins of the Human Genome Project (HGP) is shrouded in haze. It was originally conceived, it was thought, from America's contrite commitment to track the genetic defects resulting from the radioactive aftermath of Hiroshima and Nagasaki. When technology produced a method for the automated sequencing of DNA—a technology that Watson and Crick could have conceived of only in their wildest dreams—the sequencing of the genome, it appeared, was the best way to understand the defects caused by radiation and a national project was proposed. Even if that was the impetus, the project morphed into an amalgam of more lofty ambitions. "It would grant insight into human biology previously held only by God," as a 1987 article in the *New York Times* said.

The concept was far too tantalizing to ignore, as it could be the foundation of an ambitious new era of personalized medicine. By 1990, the planning was complete. Over a period of fifteen years, the HGP would attempt to sequence all three billion base pairs of the human genome. Nobel Prize winner and Harvard professor Walter Gilbert described it as "the biggest, costliest, most provocative biomedical research project in history."

It came as no surprise that James Watson was appointed head of the NIH faction of the HGP. He would finish what he started more than thirty-five years earlier when he discovered DNA, the molecule at the center of the biotech revolution. But he became embroiled in a controversy over whether NIH should allow the newly sequenced genes to be patented. He felt that the project should be public domain so that all could benefit. "We would not want one individual or company to monopolize the legal right to the beneficial information of a human gene—information that should be used for the betterment of the human race as a whole," he said. He lost the battle. He was forced to resign, and after some shuffling, Collins became head of the project and marshaled it to its conclusion. The HGP cost American taxpayers $3 billion—the cost of a couple of lattes from Starbucks per person.

As significant as the complete map of the genome was, perhaps the more significant achievement of the HGP was the remarkable improvement in speed and efficiency in sequencing technology over the project's span. The cost to sequence all three billion base pairs was $500 million, and it took thirteen years, two years ahead of schedule. By 2007, the technology had improved to the point where sequencing the entire genome would have cost $8.9 million. To sequence the entire genome today would cost $5,000 and take two days. Experts expect to hit the fabled "thousand-dollar" genome soon. The pace of sequencing efficiency blew away Moore's Law (the law describing the jaw-dropping pace at which computing speed increases). By 2000, with the HGP on its final lap and the sequencing machines soon to be idle, a seductive possibility emerged. *Could it be possible to sequence the genomes of cancer cells?* The thought had occurred to many. The revolution in "the diagnosis, prevention, and treatment of most, if not all, human diseases" that Clinton promised in his speech *could* begin with cancer.

In the winter of 2005, the highly anticipated announcement came. The NIH held a press conference in Washington, DC, announcing the launch of "a comprehensive effort to accelerate our understanding of the molecular basis of cancer through the application of genome analysis technologies, especially large-scale genome sequencing." The grand governmental project was called The Cancer Genome Atlas. The acronym TCGA was created by using the base pair abbreviations of the genetic code.

The TCGA consortium was organized and consisted of groups spanning labs in multiple nations. Another lab, funded by private money and headed by Bert Vogelstein at Johns Hopkins University, worked parallel to the government funded project, complementing rather than competing with the consortium.

"Is It Possible to Make Sense Out of This Complexity?"

Born in 1949, Vogelstein was quiet and distant as a child. He liked to skip school and retreat to the library where he immersed himself in science fiction books. He was a brilliant mathematician, and his university professors convinced him to study mathematics in graduate school.

But he soon realized that he wanted to make an impact on people's lives on a visceral level, so he switched paths and went to medical school at Johns Hopkins University, where he graduated in 1974. He discovered that his true passion was medical research. He loved the mystery and the search. He was so good at it that he became the head of one of the best funded and most productive cancer research laboratories in the country. The productivity of his lab comes from his leadership. He does not rule his laboratory but guides it like a master conductor. His students are, like him, motivated by the art of discovery and the feeling that their work has profound meaning. He created an environment for his coworkers to flourish. Well aware that the creative process is intertwined with an uninhibited mindset, he had ping-pong tables installed in his lab and started a band with his coworkers. Unassuming and humble, he makes people feel at ease. In addition to his charming nature, one is also struck by how his mind works. He thinks like a mathematician; numbers, probabilities, correlations, patterns, relationships, symmetry, and asymmetry.

His rising star was sparked when his laboratory identified the importance of p53 mutations in cancer. P53 was the most commonly mutated gene in all cancers, mutated in over 50 percent of cases. It was the poster child of oncogenes.

In 2003, Vogelstein was ranked as the most highly cited scientist in the world during the previous twenty years, according to the Institute for Scientific Information. The number of awards, and the money showered on him, were stunning. He was among eleven scientists named the first winners of the world's richest academic prize for medicine and biology. The Breakthrough Prize in Life Sciences awarded $3 million per recipient, more than twice the amount of the Nobel Prize. It was established by four Internet entrepreneurs: Yuri Milner, a Russian entrepreneur and philanthropist; Sergey Brin, cofounder of Google; Anne Wojcicki, the founder of the genetics company 23andMe and Brin's wife; and Facebook founder Mark Zuckerberg. Wojcicki told *The Times* that the prize was meant to reward scientists "who think big, take risks and have made a significant impact on our lives."

Perhaps more than anyone throughout the nineties and into the new millennium, Vogelstein shaped the image of cancer as a genetic disease, clarifying the ephemeral border of cancer's genetics. And in

2006, as the massive sequencing machines sprang to life, beginning their mission to construct cancer's bold new atlas, Vogelstein became the voice of the colossal project whether he asked for it or not.

With the funding in place and the consortium and Vogelstein's team ready to go, the sequencing of cancer genomes began in the fall of 2006. As the results began to trickle in, and then came more quickly, researchers anxiously analyzed the data, looking for mutational fingerprints that were responsible for a given type of cancer.

The stage was set for what researchers had expected to see decades earlier. Doctors like George Papanikolaou (who developed the Pap smear) and others noticed that cancer didn't just appear but underwent a predictable, step-by-step trek toward malignancy. Long before the malignant form of cervical cancer occurred, Papanikolaou noticed populations of premalignant cells burst through the confines of normal growth restraints. Although they were not yet invasive, it was easy to tell that they were well on the way.

During the eighties and nineties, inspired by the observation, Vogelstein set out to match the graded series of steps observed in the clinic to genetic alteration, thereby tying cause to effect. He focused on colon cancer, because like cervical cancer, clinicians noticed that it had a graded progression, sometimes taking decades before reaching the advanced, invasive stage. Vogelstein collected samples from patients representing four distinct stages of progression. He screened the samples for mutations. Although the technology was not yet available to screen the samples for all mutations, what he found hinted that each stage matched with a certain genetic lesion. Mutations marched lockstep with clinical progression. An orderly pattern of the mutational process emerged out the work. It was a theoretically pleasing idea that merged perfectly with the current theory of cancer. Vogelstein demonstrated that cancer was, in all probability, a step-by-step process driven by a progressive series of mutations. Not only was cancer intelligible on the level of mutation, but it also displayed a temporal pattern, moving through time in definable steps. Vogelstein painted an image of cancer as an orderly disease, one that could be understood. That was what researchers expected to see as the data from TCGA poured in: "Vogelstein-like" models for each form of cancer, a tidy sequence of mutations, a distinctive signature defining the transformation from normal cell to killing cell.

As the data from TCGA were analyzed, researchers quickly realized that a tidy series of mutations simply wasn't there, even though Vogelstein's model suggested that was what they should see. More alarming, the data failed to reveal any sort of consistent pattern. It contained a degree of randomness that caught everyone by surprise. Cancer was always characterized by its complexity, but researchers thought that at the fundamental level of mutation, chaos would turn to clarity and understanding would prevail. Over a century of work had led to this moment, all of it collapsing on the dogmatic belief that cancer was a genetic disease. Just as it appeared that the tide was turning in the researchers' favor and they would know cancer in its entirety—one year into the largest government project ever to elucidate the nature of the disease—cancer changed the rules. It took what they thought they knew about the genetics of cancer and scattered it into the wind.

To appreciate the situation cancer biology was in, you had to walk through the data from the TCGA. The implications and consequences of the data were enormous.

In 2006, Vogelstein's lab published the results from the first large-scale effort to systematically screen individual tumors from breast and colon cancer samples for somatic mutations. The results contained the first surprise: remarkably few previously unknown oncogenes were identified. It was assumed that new key oncogenes would be identified, but no one could be sure how many. That was not to be the case. Maybe the decades of work teasing out oncogenes in labs like

Vogelstein's and Weinberg's had been more thorough than researchers realized.

The initial studies were relatively limited in that they did not
sequence the twenty thousand genes contained in the human genome.
The more comprehensive studies to come revealed more. In 2007,
Vogelstein's lab sequenced samples from breast and colon cancer.
These studies delved further into the genomes of these cancers than
previous work, hoping to cull out the handful of genes behind these
common types of cancer. Like before, when the results were published,
that was not the case.

No new oncogenes were found, but far more unsettling than that
was the realization that none of the mutations found were conclusively
determined to be responsible for the origin of the disease. For the SMT
to work, mutational patterns had to be found that explained the origin
of a given type of cancer—cause must precede and explain effect. The
step-by-step series of mutations weren't there. The mutations determined to start and drive the disease were vastly different from person
to person. The degree of difference in mutations is called *intertumoral
heterogeneity*. It is a quantification of variability. If ten colon cancer
samples extracted from different patients were all found to contain
the same oncogenes A, B, D, and F, the degree of intertumoral heterogeneity is zero, because all the samples contained the same mutations. But if, for example, sample 1 contained oncogenes A, B, D, and
F, and sample 2 contained oncogenes M, R, Q, K, and Y, and sample 3
contained just oncogene Z, and so on, then the degree of intertumoral
heterogeneity is high, because the oncogenes are very different from
sample to sample.

The high degree of intertumoral heterogeneity revealed by TCGA
shocked everyone. No single mutation could be identified that was
required for the disease to start. No combination of mutations that initiated the disease could be found. Other than a few commonly mutated

oncogenes, there was a frightening degree of randomness. The studies sequenced the tumors from eleven individuals with breast cancer and eleven individuals with colon cancer. Over eighteen thousand genes were sequenced, almost forty times the number in the initial studies and the most exhaustive sequencing to date. Vogelstein was stunned by the seeming random nature of the cancer genome seen two years into the project. He posed the question on everybody's mind: "Is it possible to make sense out of this complexity?"

The sequencing technology continued to improve, becoming faster, cheaper, and more accurate. The consortium—armed, reinvigorated, and determined—took on pancreatic cancer next. In 2008, Vogelstein's group sequenced more than twenty thousand genes, nearly all of the predicted protein coding genes in the human genome, from the tumors of twenty-four individuals suffering from pancreatic cancer. It was more of the same. No new mutations of any significance were found, and the mutations they did find could not be assigned as definitely causative. Like the studies of colon and breast cancer, a shocking degree of intertumoral heterogeneity was revealed. A modification was needed to make the SMT continue to work.

A Paradigm Shift

Vogelstein knew that the SMT was in trouble. Enough data were compiled to determine that his model of a series of sequential mutations as the cause of cancer could be scrapped. He tweaked the original theory, proclaiming that rather than a defined set of specific mutations being the cause of a given cancer, cancer was caused by mutations that rendered certain biological systems dysfunctional (those involved in the qualitative aspects of cancer like uncontrolled proliferation, inhibition of programmed cell death, and tissue invasion). Cancer, Vogelstein reasoned, must be a cellular systems disease. A given system might need twenty or so constituent genes for it to operate, or so the theory went. If one constituent gene was rendered dysfunctional by a mutation, the whole system was made nonoperational, thrusting the cell one step closer to malignancy. The clutch in a car needed many parts to make the whole system work, but if one part was broken, the entire clutch system was nonoperational.

A minority of cancer biologists claimed that this was an ad hoc modification necessary to make a failed theory fit the data. For sure it was a broadening or a dilution of definition; for sure it would make the data easier to fit. Others argued that calling cancer a "systems disease" made perfect sense. The cell does operate through complex systems, and cancer could be categorized as a disease of systems gone awry, but the data would have to validate it.

Concerning the 2008 pancreatic cancer study Vogelstein wrote this about the SMT paradigm shift: "From an intellectual viewpoint, the pathway perspective helps bring order and rudimentary understanding to a very complex disease." Applying the modified theory to the study determined that pancreatic cancer was caused by the dysfunction of twelve different biological systems. A critical eye was cast on how diluted this modified theory had become. In this case it appeared to have been pretty watered down. It turned out the authors had to use some imagination to assign some of the mutations to one of the twelve systems implicated in the pathogenesis of pancreatic cancer. It appeared that some of the mutated genes were "friends of a friend of a friend" of a gene that was part of the implicated system. By the authors' own admission, "we cannot be certain that every identified mutation plays a functional role in the pathway or process in which it is implicated." Rather than bringing order to a complex disease, it seemed like the authors may, to some degree, have been manufacturing it.

Despite the confusion, TCGA soldiered on. In the fall of 2008, Vogelstein's lab published the results of sequencing glioblastoma multiforme (GBM), an aggressive form of brain cancer. Teams of researchers sequenced more than twenty thousand genes from twenty-two tumor samples. A novel oncogene was found to be mutated in 12 percent of the samples, and Vogelstein's team cited the discovery as a "validation of the utility of genome-wide genetic analysis of tumors." The results concluded that GBM was caused by mutations that rendered three core biological systems dysfunctional. However, like pancreatic cancer, a close look at the data revealed something else. None of the studies were able to validate the SMT of cancer, not even the new modified systems version, and none were able to conclude that mutations were the cause of the disease at all. Of the twenty-two samples, only four had mutations involving all three systems implicated as necessary for GBM to occur. Nine samples had mutations in two of the three systems, five had mutations in one of the three, and most significant, one sample (sample labeled Br20P) had no mutations in any of the three systems and yet was an aggressive case of GBM. The silence with regard to these inconsistencies in the new and modified SMT of cancer was striking. For the original theory or the new theory to work, samples like Br20P could not exist.

In 2013, the sequencing data on more than twenty-one thousand genes from one hundred breast cancer samples, the most comprehensive to date, were released. And for the SMT of cancer, it was the most damning to date. The authors paid homage to the complexity of the sequencing data, declaring, "The panorama of mutated cancer genes and mutational processes in breast cancer is becoming clearer, and a sobering perspective on the complexity and diversity of the disease is emerging. Driver mutations are operative in many cancer genes. A few are commonly mutated, but many infrequently mutated genes collectively make a substantial contribution in myriad different combinations."

That statement did not approach a realistic description of the complexity found in the mutation profile of breast cancer or most types of cancer. From the one hundred samples sequenced, forty-four genes were implicated as being involved in the tumorigenesis of breast cancer. The maximum number of mutated cancer genes in an individual breast cancer was six, but twenty-eight cases showed only a single driver mutation. That statement is worth repeating: *twenty-eight cases showed only a single driver mutation.* The data flew in the face of everything predicted by the SMT of cancer. Vogelstein's model, proclaiming that the hallmark features of cancer were acquired by a progressive series of mutations, did not account for the existence of a mature cancer with a single driving mutation, yet there it was.

Much worse, in another glaring omission, the authors failed to mention five samples that had no mutations at all. No driver mutations were found, yet like sample Br20P, these were living, aggressive killer cancer cells, histologically identical to the other samples. Again, for the SMT of cancer to work, samples like these couldn't exist. Embedded within the sample was the implication that something other than mutations was initiating and driving the disease.

Four years into the project, it was time to pause and reflect on the data. In 2010, Larry Loeb of the University of Washington and his colleagues attempted to summarize what had been learned so far in a review titled, "Mutational Heterogeneity in Human Cancers: Origin and Consequences." Loeb addressed the elephant in the room: "For some, the surprise has been the unexpectedly large number and diversity of mutations present in human tumors." He put his finger on the heart of the issue. It was clear that the intertumoral heterogeneity, or the variability in mutations from sample to sample, was the most poignant feature of the disease. Each person's tumor was almost as unique as a fingerprint, as a snowflake.

Loeb also noticed a stumbling block at the starting gate. He noticed that the rate of spontaneous mutations known to strike human DNA didn't correlate with the known rate of cancer occurrence. It turns out the rate of spontaneous mutation is remarkably low. Mutations are rare and infrequent events. In addition, the cell, over eons, developed elaborate and exquisitely robust mechanisms to prevent and repair mutations to DNA. So far "more than one hundred DNA repair genes have been identified," Loeb said. The cell has a rich armament consisting of legions of repair proteins, with overlapping duties, whose sole purpose is to scan the landscape of the genome and ensure its fidelity, tirelessly, over and over again. According to Loeb's calculations, few mutations slip through the cell's repair systems. This presents a conundrum for the SMT of cancer. Puzzled by the low mutation rate yet high rate of human cancer, Loeb asked a vital question: "Thus if cancer requires as many as twelve different mutations to arise...and the mutations rate is as low as calculated...how can cancer possibly occur within the human lifetime?" To answer the question, researchers were forced to propose a new hypothesis.

For cancer to arise at all, maybe the first mutation had to be in a gene responsible for DNA repair, thus reducing the cell's capacity to prevent future mutations. A lucky shot that increased the likelihood other mutations would fail to be repaired and would "stick." The theory allowed for the *possibility* that cancer originated through the mutational process. Others argued against this idea with simple logic. If mutational events were so rare, why would a cell be more prone to mutations in the genes that evolved to prevent them? As one researcher said, "It would be like hiring corrupt bank tellers."

Even if Loeb couldn't explain how the mutational process could result in cancer, he revealed a chilling insight about the therapeutic consequences born from the vast intertumoral heterogeneity uncovered by TCGA. Because mutations varied so much from patient to patient, Loeb noticed that there was not a consistent therapeutic target. How could pharmaceutical chemists zero in on a given cancer when the target was so different from person to person? "To synthesize and test enough small molecule inhibitors to combat even half of only the kinase class of suspected tumor drivers would be a daunting undertaking on a scale that is arguably beyond our current drug-developing and regulatory capacities." Loeb painted a bleak picture. Not only was it difficult to account for the origin of cancer due to the degree of intertumoral heterogeneity and the known mutation rate, but targeting the mutations, once they had established themselves may be an exercise in futility. Loeb summarized what the data showed: "There are enormous numbers of mutations present in each tumor—and it is very, very difficult to determine which ones are causative. We do not have an adequate armament of effective drugs to target the spectrum of mutant genes within individual tumors. The mutational complexity found in cancer is truly daunting."

Like Loeb, Vogelstein knew that the bewildering genetic complexity had to be addressed. In his 2013 review, he addressed the problems with TCGA data. He explained that genomic-wide sequencing technology was far from perfect and had been shown to have a false-negative error rate from 15–37 percent. However, even taking into account the potential error rate, the data still didn't draw a tangible line between cause and effect. Another explanation was needed, and Vogelstein offered one in a section titled "dark matter."

In the 1930s, it was noticed that the orbital velocities of galaxies, including our own Milky Way, didn't make sense. Galaxies were rotating much faster than predicted by classic Newtonian mechanics. Something that could not be seen was at work. The explanation came in the postulated existence of an invisible material termed "dark matter," an ephemeral, undetected material that was influencing the universe around us. Physicists still hunt for this material today. Forty miles from my home is the latest incarnation of this eighty-year search for dark matter. In an abandoned goldmine in the Black Hills of South Dakota, a colossal effort is underway to build the detectors necessary to capture one of these elusive particles and further our understanding of the universe.

Vogelstein borrowed the term *dark matter* from astrophysics and applied it to the gaping hole in understanding revealed by TCGA. He was aware that some nebulous, presumptive process was driving cancer beyond fixed mutations. It was preventing the complete picture of cancer from being realized. He asked,

> In pediatric tumors such as medulloblastomas, the number of driver gene mutations is low (zero to two). In common adult tumors—such as pancreatic, colorectal, breast, and brain cancers—the number of mutated driver genes is often three to six, but several tumors have only one or two driver mutations. How can this be explained, given the widely accepted notion that tumor development and progression require multiple, sequential genetic alterations acquired over decades? Where are these missing mutations?

He postulated that the answer was hidden in cancer's version of dark matter. Researchers had their work cut out for them. To understand the origin of cancer, dark matter had to be revealed. What it was, or where it was, was only a guess.

As sobering as the intertumoral heterogeneity revealed by the TCGA project was, and Vogelstein's missing mutations were, a new technology exposed a quality of cancer even more sobering yet. TCGA spawned the next generation of sequencing technology: machines capable of "deep sequencing." Deep sequencing does what the name implies, it extracts an unprecedented amount of information about the mutations within a single tumor from a single patient (*deep* meant that the machines teased out the exact mutations from cell to cell within the same tumor). The degree of mutational difference that exists within the same tumor, from cell to cell, is known as *intratumoral heterogeneity*. Intratumoral heterogeneity describes the "personality" of an individual tumor. A low degree of intratumoral heterogeneity implied a boring tumor with the same mutations from cell to cell; a high degree described an unpredictable, schizophrenic personality where the mutations changed markedly from cell to cell.

Deep sequencing revealed that tumors were rarely boring. Most tumors were anything but uniform (the same mutations permeating the entire expanse). Most were mosaics of stunning complexity with wildly different mutations existing from cell to cell across the breadth of the tumor. As the sequencing machines began their trek into the mutational landscape of single tumors, it became apparent that tumors were not just vastly different from person to person (intertumoral heterogeneity) but also within the same tumor (intratumoral heterogeneity).

The SMT rests on a single model describing tumor progression. Cancer is clonal in origin, according to the SMT. The word *clonal* implies that all cells within a tumor are offspring of a single cell. According to the model, cancer starts when a single cell receives its first hit to an oncogene, as time passes, the same cell eventually accumulates mutations to other oncogenes, each one pulling the cell one step closer to full-blown malignancy. As the tumor grows, offshoots from the original clone will acquire mutations of their own. And then as the offshoot cell divides and expands, a new subclonal population of cancer cells is created with a mutational signature different from the original clone. Tumors evolve and morph as they grow, smoldering masses of exponentially expanding complexity.

As you would expect, the therapeutic consequence of both intertumoral and intratumoral heterogeneity are profound, as Loeb alluded to. A tumor with a diverse population of subclones makes drug design next to impossible. A drug may target a specific mutation within a certain system, but a subclonal population of cells likely exists that contains additional mutations in the same system, rendering the drug ineffectual. A pharmaceutical chemist might be able to plug a leaky pipe only to see it spring a new leak a few inches away, and if the chemist is able to plug both leaks, a third will appear. Intratumoral heterogeneity turned drug design into "a game of Whac-A-Mole," as one reporter described it. A prominent researcher declared that intratumoral heterogeneity represented the most important clinical feature of the cancer genome and grimly described the targeted approach to cancer treatment this way: "When an old tree falls or is logged, many seedlings are poised to take grow and take its place."

The last member of the heterogeneity family is intermetastatic heterogeneity: the mutational heterogeneity observed between the cells in the primary tumor and the cells at distant sites where the tumor has metastasized. Where intratumoral heterogeneity exists across the geography of a single tumor, intermetastatic heterogeneity describes the exponential birth of generations of cancer cells with increasing mutational complexity over expanses within the body, from one location to the next. A typical metastatic lesion can have up to twenty mutations not shared by other metastatic sites within the same patient.

Beyond the obvious therapeutic significance, intratumoral and intermetastatic heterogeneity also carry theoretical significance. If the origin of cancer is sequential mutations to key oncogenes of a single cell, every tumor must carry the indelible signature of this process. The evolution of a tumor looks like a family tree. The trunk represents the founding mutations of the entire family that permeate every generation to come. If mutations were the singular event that precipitated the disease, every tumor must have a trunk representing the founding mutations—a distinctive signature anchored into every cell. As new mutations randomly strike in successive generations, the founders will hold true, permeating every cell. If a researcher could confirm cases without founding mutations, the SMT of cancer would be blown apart.

Without founding mutations, the only conclusion left was that something other than mutations, something within Vogelstein's "dark matter," would have to initiate and drive the disease. If cancer was precipitated by damaged mitochondria and mutations were largely a side effect of the disease, one might expect to find samples without a series of founding mutations that permeated the entire sample. Mutations might come after the initiation of uncontrolled growth due to damaged mitochondria. Both models of the disease, the SMT and the metabolic theory, implied that different evolutionary paths for mutations were possible. Intratumoral sequencing allowed investigators to follow cancer back through time, arriving at the tumor's very beginning, the tumors "big bang" event.

To test this, researchers had to perform a special type of sequencing. They would have to sequence samples from multiple sites within the same tumor or from different metastatic sites. A group in the United Kingdom was doing just that, sequencing samples from different locations within primary tumors, thus measuring the degree of intratumoral heterogeneity. They were also sequencing samples from metastatic sites to determine how much intermetastatic heterogeneity existed. This type of sequencing provided a moving image of cancer from the moment it was "born" through its childhood, adolescence, and maturity. This both showed the "life history" of a tumor, and as a consequence, a glimpse into the nature of its origin.

Dr. Charles Swanton's London based group was focusing on the theoretically loaded intratumoral and intermetastaic sequencing. Their work allowed investigators to get into a time machine and follow mutations back to the origin of the tumor. Swanton is passionately interested in the mutational evolution of tumors, partly because of its theoretical significance, and partly because, as he says, "if you can understand the way a tumor evolves, then you have an opportunity to get ahead of it therapeutically," he says. Swanton likened the evolution of a tumor to playing chess with a grand master in three dimensions. It is a terribly complex battle of wits.

Therapeutic consequences aside, as Swanton followed the mutations within a single tumor back to their origin, he noticed profound anomalies. He said, "I would advise you to get away from these linear models of tumor evolution, because by and large they are an oversimplification of what's happening." As Swanton followed the mutation back to the origin of the tumors he encountered some "bewildering" data. The data were not yet published, but he said that the results were "blowing our minds" and once published would "turn some heads." With respect to the exact mutational events that precipitated cancer, Swanton said, "I'm not sure we understand it—it's phenomenally complex."

In general, they found that the number of drivers that seemed to kick off the disease was much smaller than once thought. Some cases had a single driver as the "founding" or "trunk" mutation, a fact that threw an exclusively mutational origin of cancer into question and led Vogelstein to postulate dark matter. Although it was not direct evidence for the metabolic theory of cancer, it is what one would expect if the origin was metabolic and not genetic. To be sure, even by itself, the nature of intratumoral heterogeneity was an ominous discovery that added to the pile of inconsistencies that plagued the SMT.

Vogelstein wanted cancer to make sense. Like any mathematician, he wanted it to fit into a pattern and exhibit some modicum of order. With TCGA near completion, one question cut through the heart of cancer biology: how could the staggering degree of heterogeneity and the missing mutations be reconciled with an exclusive genetic origin? How was it possible to determine the cause of any type of cancer through mutations alone? He had dedicated his life to the genetics of cancer, and in the end, a tidy explanation, an explanation that would satiate a mathematician, had eluded him. He summarized the path cancer had led him down: "I agree it can be very confusing, but you try to look down from the top, you try to view the forest from the trees. I have to look at it that way, otherwise I'm lost."

He retained the sense that his work, although rife with theoretical implications, was pragmatic. "See that building over there? That is the cancer ward, and that is why we do what we do. I won't stop until that building is emptied out." Because of this sense of mission, he switched the focus of his lab from basic sequencing to the clinical application of early diagnosis. "We have switched to early diagnosis—we think after you've sequenced five thousand cancers, you might learn a little more by sequencing another five thousand...then there comes an interesting time period where we realize, okay, we know something, we don't know everything, but when do you finally make the jump and say, okay, it's time to do something? We think we've come to that time. Maybe we haven't and we won't get anywhere, but we feel it's time to make the leap."

TCGA showed the face of cancer to be a distorted, blurry image with no borders. The mutations at the heart of the SMT of cancer had yet to fall into a predictable pattern, even within the loosened boundaries of the systems theory. The bewildering degree of intertumoral heterogeneity did not allow the origin of any type of cancer to be conclusively assigned to specific mutations. It painted cancer as a disease that changed the rules on a whim, a capricious monster that played outside the realm of cause and effect. Intratumoral heterogeneity did little to clarify the image. It displayed an image that only grew more hazy as investigators followed a tumor's "family tree" of mutations toward the original trunk. The answer lay within the nebulous realm of Vogelstein's dark matter. It alone held the answer to the origin of cancer, but what would researchers find as they began to illuminate it?

The Tortoise and the Hare

By 2010, the metabolic theory of cancer was gaining traction. For one thing, the altered metabolism of the cancer cell kept popping up in scientific journals. Whether researchers liked it or not, they couldn't ignore it.

For example, one of the most meaningful discoveries to come out of TCGA was Vogelstein's 2008 discovery of the oncogene isocitrate dehydrogenase found in 12 percent of glioblastoma cases. It is the function of the oncogene that is interesting. Isocitrate dehydrogenase is a gene that encodes one of the crucial components of oxidative energy production, linking a mutated oncogene directly to defective energy production.

There was the curious case of the drug metformin. Researchers around the world were shocked in 2006 when a retrospective study found that patients with type 2 diabetes, who were taking metformin to lower their blood sugar, had substantially reduced rates of cancer. Although the exact details of how metformin prevented cancer from developing were unknown, it was almost certainly operating through metabolism. In addition, beyond the obvious preventative measures like not smoking and avoiding other carcinogens, the only established way to reduce overall cancer rates was through caloric restriction or periodic fasting, a practice known to restore mitochondria, again linking cause to metabolism. The science was funneling researchers toward metabolism whether they liked it or not. "The reason the metabolism of cancer has had a recent rebirth is because of the discovery of genes like isocitrate dehydrogenase. P53 and KRAS (another famous oncogene) have both been linked to metabolism, and so now there are a lot of people paying attention," Vogelstein said.

Like the tortoise that caught up to the tired hare in a long-distance race, the emerging metabolic theory went far beyond Warburg's single observation and appeared to be catching up to the stumbling SMT. Others were acknowledging the blurring between the theories, and one to take notice was Weinberg.

Before 2000, beyond Virchow's loose description of cancer as pathological growth, cancer was still a faceless beast. This didn't sit well with Weinberg. In the fall of 1999, at a cancer biology conference in Hawaii, Weinberg and a colleague went hiking across a volcanic bed, and they talked about how the chaotic complexity of cancer dominated its description. Yet, they discussed, cancer was governed by rules, the disease follows a pattern and exhibits some consistent traits.

Thoughts from the Hawaiian conference swirled in Weinberg's mind in the months that followed. He reduced the complexity of cancer to six underlying principles, "hallmarks" that described the most salient features. His findings were published in 2000 in the journal *Cell*, and his hallmarks became the seminal description of cancer's personality. Today they are the backbone of every textbook written on the subject. Over a decade after the article was published it is still the most cited article ever published by the journal.

Weinberg's hallmarks were as follows: (1) cancer cells stimulate their own growth, (2) they evade growth suppressing signals, (3) they resist cell death (apoptosis), (4) they enable replicative immortality, (5) they induce the ability to grow new blood vessels enabling tumor growth (angiogenesis), and (6) they spread to distant sites (metastasis).

Just as Vogelstein's multistep model of cancer was underpinned by matching genetic mutations to clinical progression, Weinberg proposed the same idea with respect to his rules. Each rule was not a theoretical abstraction but was driven by specific mutations. And as with Vogelstein, TCGA did little to validate Weinberg's hypothesis. A recent TCGA follow-up study attempting to identify the mutations driving Weinberg's sixth hallmark of metastasis found none. *"Comprehensive sequencing was unable to find a single mutation responsible for the most important quality of cancer,* the single feature of cancer responsible for 90 percent of all cancer deaths. It's like a detective that responds to a call telling him to investigate a multiple homicide."

The analogy was as follows. When the detective arrived at a murder scene, he saw a man standing in front of a house, covered in blood and holding a knife. Once the suspect was apprehended, the detective went into the house to find blood spattering the walls and floor, furniture upturned, and victims lying where they died. But as the detective and his forensic scientists combed the scene, they were unable to find evidence linking the man holding the knife to the crime—no fingerprints, no DNA evidence, not even a single fiber. Even though it seemed obvious to the detective that the man he encountered when he arrived was responsible, at some point, the evidence forced him to entertain other possibilities.

Throughout his career, Pedersen told the cancer community that it needed to stop focusing on "the man holding the knife" and that there was an equally compelling suspect, but nobody was listening. In March 2009, he got a bigger microphone to plead his case. He was invited to give a talk at an NIH seminar highlighting his life's work on cancer. It was a fascinating talk because it built up to an amazing climax: the discovery of 3BP.

Twelve minutes into the talk, he did something uncharacteristic. The humble scientist "called out" Weinberg for omitting the Warburg effect from his list of hallmarks. He said,

The hallmarks of cancer have been listed in a very well-known book now by Bob Weinberg of MIT, and he lists six hallmarks of cancer. One of these, the first and most important one, he omitted. This broadcast I understand is being broadcast throughout the world, so he'll get this probably in the mail tomorrow...many of us are aware of the list, but the one he omitted from this list is the Warburg effect. It is the oldest known property of cancer, and it is a characteristic of every cancer.

In 2010, a year after Pedersen's public challenge, Weinberg published an article in the journal *Cell* titled "Hallmarks of Cancer: The Next Generation." As the name implied, it revisited the six hallmarks in the light of more than a decade of new research. Weinberg thought there was enough evidence to justify the addition of two new "emerging" hallmarks. The first was cancer's ability to evade destruction by the immune system. This was an important feature, even more so in light of an emerging class of drugs designed to harness the immune system to combat cancer. Weinberg called the second addition "reprogramming of energy metabolism"—another way of saying the Warburg effect.

Though Weinberg met Pedersen's call to add the Warburg effect as one of cancer's most salient features, there was a profound distinction between the way Pedersen viewed the Warburg effect and the way Weinberg viewed it. Pedersen believed that cancer cells were forced to ferment glucose even in the presence of oxygen because they had to. Their mitochondria were either damaged or missing. Warburg believed the same before Pedersen and others provided substantial evidence to show how broken the mitochondria of the cancer cell were.

Weinberg didn't see it that way. He made no mention of mitochondria in his new hallmark features. The name he chose for the second emerging hallmark, "reprogramming of energy metabolism," revealed how he viewed the Warburg effect. He saw it as coming from the nucleus—a reprogramming of metabolism driven by oncogenes. He maintained that a functional reason for the Warburg effect remained "elusive" but that it was another quality of a cancer cell "programmed by proliferation-inducing oncogenes." Both sides agreed that the Warburg effect was important, but they disagreed on its cause.

Part 5

Watson Reconsiders

During the sweltering heat in August of 2009, Wall Street was in the middle of a once-in-a-century financial crisis that evoked real fears of the next Great Depression, and a gloomy anxiety engulfed the city. But James Watson wasn't feeling it. In fact, the iconic eighty-one-year-old seemed to be percolating with optimism.

Something had inspired him to write an op-ed for the *New York Times* titled "To Fight Cancer, Know the Enemy." He boldly declared, "Beating cancer now is a realistic ambition." In an even bolder gesture, he put a clock to the goal, declaring that researchers were on track to develop "lifelong cures within a decade." What could have possibly led to Watson's new found optimism? This was an abrupt about-face. He wasn't predisposed to optimism. He had experienced a lifetime of transcendental moments of hope in the war against cancer when it seemed that the tide might be shifting—all of them decisively crushed by the impenetrable force of the disease. Grand prognostications declaring an imminent cure—of the sort he just made—littered the road of cancer's arc through history.

Halfway into the article, the "father of DNA" made a surprising suggestion. Specifically, he suggested that researchers around the world should shift their focus from the genetics to the metabolism of cancer. He stated,

> While targeted combination chemotherapies would be a big step forward, I fear we still do not yet have in hand the "miracle drugs" that acting alone or in combination would stop most metastatic cancer cells in their tracks. To develop them, we may have to turn our main research focus away from decoding the genetic instructions behind cancer and toward understanding the chemical reactions (metabolism) within cancer cells.

The genetic bedlam revealed by TCGA had to be part of the shift. Even if researchers were convinced that cancer had an exclusively genetic origin, the random nature of driver mutations—not to mention intratumoral heterogeneity—made drug design brutally difficult if not impossible. Watson must have had some sort of an epiphany to call for a return to the bygone era when biochemists reigned supreme—the age of Warburg, Lehninger, Pedersen, and others.

Watson wrote,

> In the late 1940s, when I was working toward my doctorate, the top dogs of biology were its biochemists who were trying to discover how the intermediary molecules of metabolism were made and broken down. After my colleagues and I discovered the double helix of DNA, biology's top dogs then became its molecular biologists, whose primary role was finding out how the information encoded by DNA sequences was used to make the nucleic acid and protein components of cells. Clever biochemists must again come to the fore to help us understand the cancer cell chemically as well as we do genetically.

Researchers couldn't help but wonder what had inspired his epiphany. Was it TCGA or something else? The timing was telling. Ko had just sent him the data on 3BP, almost the same time as the tense Manhattan lunch date. Something compelling must have caught his eye, or he would not have combined the new strategic focus on metabolism with the bold prognostication for "real cures for most if not all cancers...within the decade" (especially during the throes of the largest governmental effort conceived and dedicated to understanding the genetic origin of cancer).

The claim that Lewis Cantley—the Cantley to whom Watson had given Ko's 3BP data—and his coworkers had discovered the significance of the Warburg effect was embedded in the article. For Watson to make the leap from Warburg to Cantley was to ignore Pedersen's lifetime of work. Watson wrote,

The idea that cancer cells may be united in having a common set of molecules not found in most other cells of our bodies was first proposed by the great German biochemist Otto Warburg. In 1924, he observed that all cancer cells, irrespective of whether they were growing in the presence or absence of oxygen, produce large amounts of lactic acid. Yet it wasn't until a year ago that the meaning of Warburg's discovery was revealed: The metabolism of cancer cells, and indeed of all proliferating cells, is largely directed toward the synthesis of cellular building blocks from the breakdown products of glucose. This discovery indicates that we need bold new efforts to see if drugs that specifically inhibit the key enzymes involved in this glucose breakdown have anti-cancer activity.

To those aware of Pedersen's body of work, Watson's claim that Cantley had recently discovered the meaning behind the Warburg effect seemed misguided. Pedersen had spent more than thirty years mapping out detailed descriptions of the why and the how of the Warburg effect. The pathway was part of the Warburg effect but by no means the entire story. Watson's call for "clever biochemists to again come to the fore" was what Pedersen had been saying all along. But the statement had been made. To those paying attention, Watson's call for all troops to change strategy was shocking. Any call to move resources away from the dogma of targeted drug design, especially from someone as respected as Watson, represented a monumental moment in the annals of cancer.

Others did not share Watson's optimism. In the years surrounding his 2009 op-ed, cancer had returned to the public eye. Steve Jobs's death in 2011 thrust the disease into the media spotlight. The fact that the man who epitomized technological progress was lost to cancer was symbolic of the disease's unbreakable trajectory and how it mocked our efforts to control it. David Agus, the prominent oncologist who treated Jobs, was even booed during a speech given after Job's death when Agus suggested that we might just have to learn to treat cancer without understanding it—a capitulation to the complexity of the disease. Others shared Agus's frustration. It seemed that a collective boiling point had been reached, in part, because the numbers dug up by journalists were abysmal.

The national attempt to beat cancer, kicked off by Nixon, had been a failure, and journalists were taking notice. The statistics were everywhere. If you were a woman, you had a one in three chance of being diagnosed with cancer in your lifetime. If you were a man, your chances were one in two. Within the next decade, cancer was likely to replace heart disease as the leading cause of death, according to forecasts by NCI and the Center for Disease Control and Prevention (CDC). In a 2004 *Fortune* article titled "Why We're Losing the War on Cancer," Clifton Leaf wrote,

It is already the biggest killer of those under 75. Among those ages 45 to 64, cancer is responsible for more deaths than the next three causes—heart disease, accidents, and stroke—put together. It is also the leading killer of children, thirtysomethings—and everyone in between.

The most important statistic, the one that told the story with the most unbiased clarity, was that the current death rate from cancer was still the same as it was in 1950.

Siddhartha Mukherjee released *The Emperor of All Maladies: A Biography of Cancer* in 2010, a book that *Time* rated as one of the one hundred most important books since 1923 (the year the magazine was founded). In the summer of 2013, Leaf—a cancer survivor, former *New York Times* guest editor, and acclaimed author—released *The Truth in Small Doses: Why We Are Losing the War on Cancer and How to Win It*. That same summer, science writer George Johnson released *The Cancer Chronicles: Unlocking Medicine's Deepest Mystery*, which he wrote after the woman he loved was diagnosed with metastatic cancer. The authors of all these books explored every nuance of our history with, and effort to combat the disease. All three were inspired by how much we don't know and how ineffectual our attempts at treatment have been. One decade into the twenty-first century, it was clear that the promise of TCGA had taunted us with hope only to violently jerk it out of our reach. A common theme was emerging. Every article or book written on the subject led the reader down the same path as TCGA, capitulating that the failure was the result of the way that cancer scrambled mutations into an unbreakable code.

In the winter of 2013, one day after the annual report to the nation compiled by a coalition of some of the country's top cancer organizations on the status of cancer was released, Watson released his own article in the journal *Open Biology* titled "Oxidants, Antioxidants, and the Current Incurability of Metastatic Cancers." It was the culmination of months of work that he described as "among my most important work since the double helix." The article reflected the nation's state of mind and was a brutal assessment of the ongoing war. It did not shy away from harsh criticisms and again called for a complete refocusing of direction. Watson wrote,

> *Even though we will soon have comprehensive views of how most cancers arise and function at the genetic and biochemical level, their "curing" seems now to many seasoned scientists an even more daunting objective than when the "War on Cancer" was started by President Nixon in December 1971.*

It read like an eruption of frustration, but it resonated with the national mood at the time. The article merged with the spate of books, articles, and newscasts revisiting the failed war against cancer, a gloominess that seemed to infect the collective consciousness. Jedidiah Becker for redOrbit.com wrote, "Although no doubt unwelcomed in many quarters of the research community, Watson's report comes at a time when even the most ardent devotees of the cancer research establishments are growing increasingly disheartened over the meager progress being made by current approaches to cancer treatment."

How meager had the progress been? A close look at the next generation of targeted drugs conceived out of decades of work prior to and from TCGA exposed what a dismal failure the approach has been. The public was realizing that promises were unfulfilled. Watson capitulated to this realization, saying, "The now much-touted genome-based personal cancer therapies may turn out to be much less important tools for future medicine than the newspapers of today led us to believe."

A look at the numbers confirmed his assessment. Since Herceptin kicked off the targeted drug revolution, an objective look at the results painted a depressing picture. "A conservative estimate of the number of targeted therapies tested in patients with cancer in the past decade was seven hundred," said Antonio Tito Fojo, PhD, head of the Experimental Therapeutics Section and senior investigator for Medical Oncology Branch Affiliates at the Center for Cancer Research at the National Cancer Institute in Bethesda, Maryland, "yet no patients with solid tumors have been cured by targeted therapies over that time period. Zero [is] the number of targeted therapies that have prolonged survival by one year, when compared to a conventional treatment." Science writer Ralph Moss noticed the odd criteria that the FDA used to approve drugs that allowed scores of ineffectual drugs to gain approval:

If you can shrink the tumor 50 percent or more for 28 days you have got the FDA's definition of an active drug. That is called a response rate, so you have a response...(but) when you look to see if there is any life prolongation from taking this treatment what you find is all kinds of hocus pocus and song and dance about the disease free survival, and this and that. In the end there is no proof that chemotherapy in the vast majority of cases actually extends life, and this is the GREAT LIE about chemotherapy, that somehow there is a correlation between shrinking a tumor and extending the life of the patient.

An example of the current state of cancer drugs is bevacizumab (Avastin). It received FDA approval in 2004 for metastatic colon cancer and later received approval for other applications including breast cancer. To treat the average breast cancer patient with Avastin cost $90,816 per year without extending overall survival. But because it shrank tumors in a fraction of cases, the FDA approved it, highlighting the absurd criteria used for drug approval. Worse, patients who were treated with Avastin on top of paclitaxel had double the chance of experiencing significantly higher toxicity. Doctors must have realized the contradiction when recommending Avastin. Did they really tell patients that they should take a full course of the drug but would likely experience two and a half times the normal toxicity? The drug cost almost $100,000, and it wouldn't extend life at all. Why would an oncologist prescribe it? "There is a shocking disparity between value and price, and it's not sustainable," said Roy Vagelos, MD, at the 2008 annual meeting of the International Society for Medical Publication Professionals.

The cost-benefit relationship for almost every one of these drugs was marginal at best and nonexistent at worst. The cost for cancer drugs went from an average of about $5,000 before 2000 to $40,000 by 2005, and in 2012, almost every new drug was priced at more than $100,000 in the United States. The United States spent twice as much as any other country on oncology and medical care in general yet achieved the same survival rate except for breast cancer and lymphoma, where it eked out a 1–2 percent better survival rate.

In four years, Watson went from declaring "lifelong cures within a decade" to an "even more daunting objective" today than when Nixon made his famous declaration almost forty years ago. The numbers backed up what he was saying, and the science gave an explanation. Even if researchers insisted that cancer was purely a genetic disease, both the intertumoral and intratumoral heterogeneity revealed by TCGA forced them to admit that cancer put their attempts to therapeutically target mutations in checkmate. From a genetic perspective, it seemed that the more researchers learned of it, the more it appeared incurable. Watson must have known this, because like Vogelstein, he declared that it was time to move on. "While I initially supported TCGA getting big monies, I no longer do so. Further 100 million dollar annual injections so spent are not likely to produce the truly break-through drugs that we so desperately need," Watson wrote.

If it was time to move on, what was it time to move on to? If the purported origin of cancer, mutations to DNA, gave no hope for a cure, what could? Vogelstein moved on, but he wasn't developing therapies. He had moved on to early diagnosis. If cancer put drug designers in a therapeutic checkmate, he reasoned that maybe doctors could front run the disease. Early detection still offered far and away the best prognosis for those diagnosed.

Watson had other ideas. As in his op-ed in 2009, he circled back to the metabolism of cancer: "We must focus much, much more on the wide range of metabolic and oxidative vulnerabilities [of cancer cells]." He then mentioned 3BP when he wrote, "3-bromopyruvate, the powerful dual-inhibitor of hexokinase as well as oxidative phosphory-lation, kills highly dangerous hepatocellular carcinoma cells and so has the capacity to truly cure, at least in rats, an otherwise highly incurable cancer." It appeared that he was ready to walk away from his molecule and spend more time looking at the biochemistry of the cancer cell that Warburg identified more than eighty years earlier.

Once showered with superlatives, TCGA was thought to be the final chapter that would lead to a complete understanding of can-cer followed by real and enduring cures. Now almost a decade old, it seemed as though the project had only stirred up a cloud of con-fusion and left a trail of unfulfilled promises in is wake. Watson and Vogelstein, the two who embodied the spirit of the project perhaps more than anyone, were leaving it behind.

Part 6

Mitochondria: An Old Theory Is New Again

It is good for the entire enterprise that mitochondria and chloroplast have remained small, conservative, and stable, since these two organelles are, in a fundamental sense, the most important living things on the earth. Between them they produce the oxygen and arrange for its use. In effect, they run the place.

My mitochondria comprise a very large proportion of me. I cannot do the calculation, but I suppose there is almost as much of them in sheer dry bulk as there is the rest of me. Looked at in this way, I could be taken for a very large, motile colony of respiring bacteria, operating a complex system of nuclei, microtubules, and neurons for the pleasure and sustenance of their families, and running, at the moment a typewriter.

I am intimately involved, and obliged to do a great deal of essential work for my mitochondria. My nuclei code out the outer membranes of each, and a good many of the enzymes attached to the cristae must be synthesized by me. Each of them, by all *counts, makes only enough of its own materials to get along on, and the rest must come from me. And I am the one who has to do the worrying.*

Now that I know about the situation, I can find all kinds of things to worry about. Viruses, for example. If my organelles are really symbiotic bacteria, colonizing me, what's to prevent them from catching a virus, or if they have such a thing as lyogeny, from conveying a phage to other organelles? Then there is the question of my estate. Do my mitochondria all die with me, or did my children get some of mine along with their mother's; this sort of thing should not worry me, I know, but it does.

— From The Lives of a Cell, by Lewis Thomas
The Prologue of Pete Pedersen's 1978 review
"Tumor Mitochondria and the Bioenergetics of
Cancer Cells"

The importance of mitochondria predates everything human, mammal, reptile, amphibian, or dinosaur. Evolution's march up the ladder of complexity may not have been possible if not for an accidental, fortuitous event that gave existence to mitochondria.

To understand mitochondria, we have to understand symbiosis, another feature pervasive to life. All life engages in "I'll rub your back if you rub mine" behavior. We inhale what plants exhale and vice versa. We need each other. One cannot exist without the other. Humans have ten times as many bacteria in the gut than cells in the entire body. They manufacture vitamins, train the immune system, and keep pathogenic bacteria at bay. Everywhere we look on the planet, life is engaged in a symphony of cooperation. One scientist described life's penchant for symbiosis by saying, "Life did not take over the globe by combat but by networking." Mitochondria are no different. They once existed as a separate entity outside of cells as free-living bacteria. Then, through some twist of fate, the bacterium was taken inside of another cell and incorporated as an endosymbiont.

The relationship proved to be advantageous for both. Over time the once-separate entities begin to cooperate. The bacterium found it was best to concentrate on producing energy and agreed to transfer most of its genome to the host cell's DNA, leaving the host cell to specialize in the storage of information and the organization of the cell overall. The relationship, lavishly interconnected over the course of millennia, blurred the distinction between the two. Today, the nuclear genome has incorporated, or developed, approximately three thousand mitochondrial genes, leaving the mitochondria responsible for only twenty-four genes within its own DNA – DNA that retains the same circular structure of bacterial DNA, reflecting the bacterial origin of mitochondria.

Mitochondria became remarkably efficient at manufacturing adenosine triphosphate (ATP), the cell's energetic "currency." At any given time, the human body has about nine ounces of ATP diffused throughout its trillions of cells, which is an unremarkable amount. It is the turnover that is remarkable. In one day, mitochondria turn over the body's weight equivalent in ATP; an astonishing degree of chemical churn. In return for their efficient production of energy, the cell takes care of most of the mitochondria's needs, transcribing proteins and shuttling molecules in and out of it. The two engage in continuous crosstalk and are intimately connected in their operations.

Mitochondria are so important to the fidelity of an organism that a predominant theory is called "the mitochondrial theory of aging." It contends that the condition of the mitochondria dictate the capacity of the cell to function over time. As mitochondria decline, cellular operations decline with them (just as if electricity and oil were cut off, the economy would grind to a halt). As the mitochondria lose the ability to function efficiently, the body begins the functional decline known as aging.

Mitochondria: An Old Theory Is New Again

Oxygen is a double-edged sword. While necessary for sustaining life, it is responsible for the slow erosion of mitochondria. The main source of free radical generation is within the mitochondria as energy is generated from whipping electrons through the electron transport chain, an inherently reactive process that requires oxygen. To combat free radicals, mitochondria developed an important antioxidant network consisting of glutathione, vitamin C, vitamin E, lipoic acid, uric acid, and antioxidant enzymes. They work synergistically. A deficiency in one can be compensated by the others. But as we age, this network degrades, leaving the mitochondria vulnerable to free radical assault. Researchers at the Linus Pauling Institute showed how banged up old mitochondria get. On average they lose up to half of important structural lipids, energy-shuttling compounds, and antioxidants with advanced age. Much of the body's decline with age is due to the "rusting" of mitochondria. As the mitochondria go, so does the rest of what we call ourselves.

Pedersen established that cancer cells had damaged and fewer mitochondria, proving Warburg's contention that cancer cells fermented because they had to. They were compensating for the "irreversible injuring of respiration." The question then arises: how were the mitochondria getting damaged in the first place? And most important, was Warburg right? Did damage to the mitochondria result in cancer? To answer the first question, scientists had to start from the end and work backward. They had to look at the agents that caused cancer and then at how they were doing it. This was where the SMT of cancer and the metabolic theory became tangled and one covered the other. There were instances where a few scientists untangled the two, exposing a different view and a glimpse into a disease that was anything but simple.

Pott's discovery of the first carcinogen in 1777 sent cancer researchers on a crusade to find other exogenous causes lurking around us.

From then on, it seemed that a continuous stream of environmental agents were shown to cause cancer. The list was stitched into the observation Hansemann made that the chromosomes of cancer cells were a mess, initially forming the SMT of cancer. The decades that followed revealed cancer to be a pathological version of hopscotch, a multistep process theoretically caused by a series of sequential mutations that kicked off malignancy. Carcinogens mutated DNA, resulting in defective cellular machinery and in turn causing cancer. It made perfect sense, but in 1948, an Englishman made a curious observation that ran decisively against the grain.

Cyril Darlington was born in an English cotton town in 1903. From the moment of his birth, everything about him was unconventional and contradictory. He had a poor, unhappy childhood but developed into a strikingly handsome man. He was tall and commanding, and women found him charming. He wanted to be a farmer, but when that didn't pan out, he dove into genetics and became a productive and respected scientist. His personality was no different; he adhered to rational logic but approached problems from unconventional angles. He was a brilliant scientist who had the unique ability to ignore dogma and look at issues with a fresh perspective.

Darlington's world view allowed him to look at cancer from the periphery rather than the center. When he examined how carcinogens operated, he noticed that the carcinogens most adroit at damaging nuclear DNA were not necessarily the best at causing cancer. At low doses, x-rays damaged chromosomes but failed to cause cancer. He also noticed that x-rays caused cancer only when given at high enough doses to damage the cytoplasm. This observation raised another question for Darlington: "How far does the experimental evidence enable us to distinguish between the nucleus and the cytoplasm (mitochondria) as the seat of the mutation (the mutation necessary to cause cancer)?"

Mitochondria: An Old Theory Is New Again

Even in 1948, the question was heretical. Before the discovery of DNA, chromosomes were still the number one suspect, but Darlington's discovery made a subtle distinction suggesting researchers were missing important details, suggesting that cancer had a cytoplasmic origin. The fact that he noticed the anomaly at all was amazing, considering that he was trained as a geneticist and conditioned to believe all cellular change began at the level of the chromosome. Carcinogens and x-rays damaged both mitochondria and nuclear DNA, but it took a radical thinker to detect the difference and tease out the details. It appeared that the agents better at damaging mitochondria were better at causing cancer. The idea would have merged effortlessly with Warburg's hypothesis, but nobody made the connection, and Darlington's observations faded into oblivion.

In 1978, in his groundbreaking review, Pedersen made the next curious observation and further muddied the waters on how carcinogens "caused" cancer. In *The Lives of a Cell* Lewis Thomas jokingly stated that he worried about his mitochondria catching a virus, but Pedersen provided definitive proof that they could. Along with corroborating Darlington's work showing that a wide swath of chemical carcinogens directly damaged mitochondria, Pedersen showed that viruses could also. He provided evidence showing how viruses used the mitochondrial machinery for replication, and he referenced pictures of viral particles living within mitochondria.

In another twist of irony, Pedersen provided evidence that RSV was able to infect the mitochondria of chicken cells. This was two years after Varmus and Bishop employed the famous virus to prove the SMT through their discovery of the viral origin of cellular oncogenes. Decades after their discovery that cancer-causing viruses act by stealing genes, holding them hostage, and putting them back as oncogenes, a mutated version of the src gene had never conclusively been implicated in any cancer outside of the transforming ability of RSV.

Like the famous chicken-or-the-egg paradox, the question was which caused cancer first: Rous's viral src gene (as Varmus and Bishop contended) or the Rous viruses' ability to infect and damage mitochondria (as Pedersen suggested)? Investigators knew that many viruses were capable of causing cancer, but not all of them inserted oncogenes directly into the DNA like RSV. The three common transforming agents—chemical carcinogens, radiation, and viruses, as Pedersen and Darlington showed—were capable of damaging both mitochondria and nuclear DNA, a fact that tangled Warburg's theory and SMT, blurring the lines between the two.

As the last decades of the twentieth century passed, evidence for a genetic origin of cancer piled up. When the technology became available to sequence the entire genome of cancer cells, the end was in sight. When TCGA began, it was the beginning of the end. Every subtle nuance of cancer would be illuminated, but it wouldn't be that simple. Cancer had another hand to play.

For scientists focused on the origin of cancer, the existence of Vogelstein's dark matter exposed a gaping hole of understanding and opened the door for new theories on the events that led to cancer. It wasn't announced on the nightly news or any large-scale media outlet. The further one extended from those at the center of the research, the less was known about the sudden and drastic change in cancer biology. For most of the scientists aware of the sequencing data, the standard response was something like, "Holy shit, cancer is complex. I guess we never realized how complex this disease really is." The result of examining the new data was not questioning the SMT of cancer but surrendering to a level of complexity never dreamed of. The strange data affected some in a much different way. Rather than being resigned to the complexity, it made them question a genetic origin altogether.

Dr. Thomas Seyfried fell into this category. "When I looked at the data, I made up my mind right away mutations had little to do with the origin of cancer." Around 2000, he made an accidental discovery that shifted the direction of his research toward the metabolism of cancer. The further he dug, the more befuddled he was that nobody other than Pedersen and a handful of others realized how much data supported Warburg's original hypothesis. "The more I learned, the more I thought this is ridiculous; what are we doing with this gene theory? How come more people don't know about this?"

In 1946, Seyfried was born in Flushing, New York, a northern neighborhood of Queens known today for its rich cultural and religious diversity. His father was a merchant marine who went into the paint industry and eventually owned his own retail outlet. The family lived in modest circumstances at the northern edge of town, of the mostly Irish and Italian community. His father moved the family to Brockton, Massachusetts, when Seyfried was seventeen. At the time, Brockton was the shoe manufacturing capital of the United States, so those of working age eventually found themselves in shoe mills. "I had to put the shoe boards in and out of the oven...it was a tough job."

After graduating from high school, Seyfried enrolled as a biology major at the University of New England. Upon graduation, with the Vietnam War in full swing, he found himself in a hopeless situation. "There were no jobs," he said, "no companies were willing to take a chance hiring anybody young because they thought they would put in all that investment only to have them drafted."

With few other options, he joined the army. He was shipped to Oklahoma and trained as a commander of field artillery. After a year in Germany, he was sent to Vietnam, where he was a forward observer with the infantry. "I aimed the cannons," he said of his stint in the war. "We were in the jungle, so you couldn't see, and I would often get erroneous targeting information, so my single greatest achievement was not killing any of my own men. The guy before me killed eighteen of our guys by friendly fire." While in Vietnam, he filled out a graduate school application to attend Illinois State University, which one of his undergraduate professors suggested. "I remember when I put the application into the envelope, it had dirt and mud on it from the jungle."

His tour in Vietnam came to an abrupt halt in 1971 when he was told that he was going home. "I was in a firefight in August, and then I was sitting in a classroom three weeks later." He admitted that the transition was difficult. "That first year was tough—I didn't get the best grades." After receiving his master's degree in genetics, he transferred to the University of Illinois, where he obtained a PhD in classical genetics.

He found himself drawn to biochemistry and focused on lipid research (fats). He concentrated on a class of lipids known as gangliosides that were comprised of a long carbon chain connected to a collection of circular carbohydrates. When drawn on paper, gangliosides look like a blooming flower. The beautiful molecules tend to concentrate in the outer membrane of cells where they relay signals, and because their flower-like head extends beyond the surface of the cell, they participate in cell-to-cell communication. But the complex, flourishing topology of gangliosides comes at a price: they are difficult to dispose of.

Typically, most macromolecules are broken down within specialized cellular organelles called lysosomes—bucket-shaped "trash cans" that are filled with acid. Lysosomes efficiently and continuously degrade and recycle cellular components. Because of their unwieldy size and shape, gangliosides require lysosomes to carry special enzymes to break them down. If a person inherits a mutation in one of the enzymes, then partially broken down gangliosides began to accumulate, clogging the lysosomes, eventually spilling over and accumulating in lethal amounts. The result is a rare class of disorders known as lipid storage diseases such as Tay-Sachs disease. Victims typically don't live past the age of four.

Mitochondria: An Old Theory Is New Again

Seyfried found himself more interested in the gangliosides themselves than the defective lysosomal enzymes that the lab was focusing on in Illinois, so he moved to New Haven, Connecticut, to complete a postdoc under Yale's highly regarded ganglioside expert, Robert Yu. Yu's lab possessed the latest techniques to isolate, purify, and elucidate the structure of the complex molecules. Seyfried worked on the basic science of gangliosides until, by accident, he made a curious observation.

A start-up English company had discovered a unique compound: a molecule that inhibited the formation of certain gangliosides. The company was excited by the prospect that the drug might be useful for treating lipid storage diseases, and it sent out samples for testing. Through a different laboratory, Seyfried obtained a sample of the drug and wanted to see how it might influence development of the brain. By inhibiting ganglioside production in developing embryos, the drug could map how gangliosides effected brain development, giving a glimpse into their functionality. Seyfried and his students began tinkering with the drug. They gave it to mice with tumors more out of playful curiosity than scientific investigation. To their surprise, the drug appeared to slow the growth of tumors compared to the control mice.

"We called the company and told them it looked like their drug might work on cancer—they were ecstatic," Seyfried said. To a start-up drug company, a drug active against cancer carried much more potential than one active against lipid storage diseases, and the market went from tiny to huge. Excited by the drug's potential, the company wrote Seyfried a check for $200,000 for further investigation. His lab got to work. Right away they noticed that the mice given the drug were losing weight. He instructed his students to adjust the diet of the control mice so that they lost the same amount of weight as the mice given the drug. To everybody's surprise, the tumors slowed in the control mice.

The drug was just causing the mice to lose their appetite, mimicking caloric restriction. Seyfried said, "I had to call the company back and tell them their drug didn't work. Of course they pulled the plug on the funding—why would they fund this stuff if you can get the same effect by eating less food?"

The strange results raised another question: why would restricting calories slow tumor growth? The observation made Seyfried wonder if other known anticancer drugs might be operating through the same mechanism, unknown to the developers. He began testing other drugs, and it turned out that many of them did, including ImClone's ERBITUX (the drug known from the Martha Stewart insider trading scandal). "Many of these drugs were doing nothing but making the mice lose their appetites. It was the reduced calories that had the antitumor effect." But why would reducing calories in general affect tumor growth? That question spun him away from ganglioside research and into the metabolism of cancer. "I hadn't even heard of Otto Warburg before the year 2000," he said.

Seyfried's launch into cancer research was backward by most standards. He began with a curious therapeutic observation and circled back to the basic science. His compulsion to understand why a tumor's growth was affected by metabolism immersed him in a fascinating detective story that took him back to Warburg. It led him to Pedersen's enormous body of work, especially his 1978 review, mapping out every nuance of cancer's terribly broken mitochondria, a body of work Seyfried referred to as a "masterpiece." Largely hidden from view, his search went through others like Rous and Darlington, scientists with uncommon insight. He gives enormous credit to the work of Carlos Sonnenschein and Ana Soto, saying they had compiled a "blistering attack on the gene theory of cancer. They did a magnificent job ferreting out all the old papers showing the inconsistencies of the gene theory." Seyfried said that his modern version of the metabolic theory of cancer was a collision of Pedersen's 1978 paper, the work of Sonnenschein and Soto, his own work on the damaged lipids of tumor mitochondria, his study of dietary effects on tumor growth, a massive literature search, and his background in genetics, which enabled him to evaluate data from TCGA. Until Seyfried, nobody had finished what Warburg had started: a theory that began with Warburg's first observation of aerobic fermentation and finished with Weinberg's six hallmarks of cancer. "People were saying it in various forms, but nobody probably said it as brashly as I did."

When Seyfried summarized all his research in his 2012 book, *Cancer as a Metabolic Disease*, it took some time for people to take notice, but they did. His phone began to ring, and his e-mail box began to fill. Even if the research giants in the field or the folks at NCI failed to notice, cancer patients and physician groups did. He was featured on radio shows and high-profile blogs. He received invites to speak at physician group conferences, many ending in standing ovations. He made a compelling case for a vastly different image of cancer, an image that gave reason for hope. Anecdotal cases of cancer patients employing metabolic therapies began to pop up—some with stunning results that defied all expectations and left doctors befuddled. If Seyfried's image of cancer was unable to penetrate the academic research world from the top down, it was doing it from the bottom up through patients, physicians, and the handful of academics who noticed. Like anything new, there would be critics. "When I give talks to scientists, you know, they are usually throwing stuff at you. Scientist are very critical about everything. We have to be. You know it's part of what we do—we don't give standing ovations to people."

Seyfried's biggest contribution to Warburg's theory was to pick up where Pedersen left off, with the looming question still hanging: how did injured mitochondria lead to uncontrolled proliferation? Always the humble pragmatist, Pedersen admitted as much in his 1978 review.

"Although we have learned much about the properties of tumor mitochondria and their overall relationship to the bioenergetics of cancer cells, we have failed to answer those questions which are most basic and fundamental to the cancer problem. First we have not established whether mitochondrial function...is essential to the normal to neoplastic transformation process."

When Vogelstein postulated the existence of dark matter, he suggested that the most obvious possibility is epigenetic drivers. The term *epigenetics* is used to describe all of the other influences that operated on DNA beyond the fixed genetic code. Unlike genetic code, epigenetic drivers are fluid, transient forces that influence the expression of genes. They respond to influences like nutritional status, hormones, and illness, allowing adaptation to a continuously changing environment. Epigenetic signaling is the crucial link, the process that Warburg was unable to identify, that would have tied his theory of cancer into a single, unified explanation.

While looking for the link between damaged respiration and uncontrolled growth, Seyfried proposed that chronic and persistent damage to the cell's ability to respire aerobically triggered an epigenetic signal from the mitochondria to nuclear DNA. The signal then altered the expression of a plethora of key cancer-causing oncogenes—a classic epigenetic system. Vogelstein readily admitted that epigenetics may play a much larger role in cancer than expected. One problem, he said, was that, "epigenetics just don't lend themselves well to experiments." Nevertheless, Seyfried illuminated the basic research showing the important epigenetic signaling that travels from the damaged mitochondria to the nucleus, the missing link to a complete metabolic theory of cancer.

To construct a single metabolic theory of cancer, Seyfried connected the last remaining dots. He tied injured mitochondria with uncontrolled proliferation, the pathological feature of cancer that

Mitochondria: An Old Theory Is New Again

Virchow documented more than one hundred years prior. Fortunately for Seyfried, the tangled relationship between the mitochondria and the nucleus was being sorted out. In addition to supplying the cell's energy needs, mitochondria were known to regulate many cellular functions including iron metabolism, heme and steroid synthesis, programmed cell death, and cellular division and differentiation. To do these functions, mitochondria talk constantly with the nucleus, relaying signals and materials back and forth.

Pedersen had shown that the single transition to hexokinase II drastically altered the metabolic landscape of the cell. By binding to the mitochondrial outer membrane, it turned the cells into immortal, crazed fermenters. In 2012, when Seyfried released his book, there was substantial experimental evidence showing how damaged mitochondria sent a distress signal called the retrograde response to the nucleus. The signal told the nucleus to transcribe a host of genes responsible for preparing the cell to ferment glucose in order to compensate for declining oxidative energy production.

The genes that responded to the mitochondrial distress call had foreign names: Myc, Tor, Ras, NfkB, and CHOP. But collectively they have profound consequences when turned on. Myc, a protein with global operations, acts as a transcription factor. It alone controls 15 percent of the entire genome. It affects vast swaths of the genomic landscape, turning some genes on and putting others to sleep, but when taken as a whole, it begins the process of tumorigenesis. Most of the genes turned on by damaged mitochondria sit at signaling hubs, and therefore dictate multiple operations like cell division and angiogenesis (the growth of new blood vessels to supply the tumor). Seyfried contends that if the retrograde signal was "on" chronically, as is the case when mitochondria are damaged beyond repair, trouble started.

A persistent retrograde response, in addition to ramping up the proteins necessary for a massive increase in energy creation through fermentation, would exhibit side effects like uncontrolled proliferation. A sustained retrograde response had even more dire consequences. As the response became chronic and genomic signals transitioned the cell into a different cellular architecture, the legions of proteins designated to protect and repair DNA began to stand down—drying out the moat and leaving the castle unguarded. Darlington noticed this phenomenon as far back as 1948 and wrote, "The development of unbalanced nuclei in tumors is without precedent in any living tissue. It implies a relaxation of detailed control of the nucleus which is also without precedent. And this in turn argues that the nucleus is not itself directly responsible for what is going on."

Left unprotected, the chromosomes are vulnerable to mutations by the increasing generation of free radicals from the damaged mitochondria. The timing is critical. The retrograde response comes first and then genomic instability. This single detail, the timing, is crucial, implying that the mutations thought to initiate the disease are merely a side effect. This went a long way to explain the befuddling data from TCGA, and it would explain the contradictory low mutation rate yet high cancer rate that Loeb noticed. If cancer is driven by the retrograde response, it could explain how mutations varied wildly from patient to patient and how samples with one or two mutations could exist. It implied that rather than driving cancer, mutations were just features of its personality.

According to Seyfried, the mutations at the heart of the SMT of cancer were downstream to the true cause: damaged mitochondria. They are a side effect, an epiphenomenon. The upshot is that mutations to DNA "arise as effects rather than as causes of tumorigenesis," Seyfried said. The mutations seen in the DNA of cancer cells are "red herrings" that had sent researchers on a futile hunt.

The most striking evidence that Seyfried dug up was from the late eighties: a series of uncomplicated experiments that cast remarkable conclusions. Not all experiments are created equal, some are better than others. Experiments that are technically simple by design yet offer results that answer big questions tend to leave a lasting mark in their fields.

Two groups working independently, one in Vermont and the other in Texas, performed a meticulous series of nuclear transfer experiments with shocking results. The experiments consisted of a simple transfer. Warren Schaeffer's group at the University of Vermont wondered how much control the cytoplasm (where all the mitochondria reside) had over the process of tumorigenesis. To find out they conceived of a beautiful experiment. Simply put, they took the nucleus of a cancer cell and transferred it into a healthy cell with its nucleus removed. The reconstituted cell (or recon) contained the DNA of the cancer cell, with all its supposed driver mutations, but it had the cytoplasm and mitochondria of a noncancerous cell.

The recon now had tremendous power. It alone could answer the question of who was right: Warburg or Varmus and Bishop. If mutations to DNA caused and drove cancer, the recons should be cancerous, regardless of their healthy mitochondria. But if, as Warburg, Pedersen, and Seyfried contended, the mitochondria are responsible for starting and driving cancer and mutations were largely irrelevant, the new recons should be normal, healthy cells.

The Vermont group found that when they transplanted the recon cells into sixty-eight mice, only a single mouse grew a tumor over the course of an entire year. The cells containing the mutations thought to be responsible for the disease were silenced by the healthy cytoplasm (mitochondria). But without a metabolic theory of cancer in place, or any theory that explained the results, Schaeffer's group was not sure what to think. They knew that the results contradicted the prevailing dogma, but they struggled to find an explanation that made sense.

While the Vermont group mulled over the strange results, Jerry Shay's group at the University of Texas Southwestern Medical Center in Dallas confirmed Schaeffer's results. They ran the same transfer experiment and injected the recons into ten mice. Not a single one developed a tumor, substantiating the amazing results seen in Vermont. Like Schaeffer's group, the Texas group struggled to make sense of the results. To ensure that an experimental artifact wasn't screwing up the results, Shay's group performed a set of painstaking controls. They took the nucleus of a cancer cell and transferred it into the cytoplasm of a cancer cell. They wanted to make sure that the experimental procedure itself wasn't responsible for turning the recons into normal cells. Seven out of the eight control recons remained cancerous when transferred to mice. They reversed the control and transferred normal nuclei into normal cytoplasm. None of the recons turned cancerous in the mice, confirming that the shocking results were not due to an experimental artifact.

Schaeffer's group then ran the same experiment in reverse. Instead of adding the nucleus of a cancer cell to the cytoplasm of a normal cell, they flipped the method and added the nucleus of a normal cell to the cytoplasm of a tumor cell (a whole tumor cell with its nucleus removed). If mutations to DNA caused cancer, the recons should be healthy, normal cells. However, if damage to the mitochondria, followed by a retrograde response to the nucleus, was the cause of cancer, the recons should have been cancerous. Again the results flew in the face of everything known about cancer, directly contradicting the SMT of cancer. When they transplanted the recons containing a malignant cytoplasm and a normal nucleus into newborn mice, 97 percent of the mice developed tumors.

The fact that both groups had shown that the cytoplasm of a normal cell, with normal mitochondria, could suppress cancer was one thing, and ardent devotees to the SMT may have been able to turn the other cheek on an isolated series of experiments. But when Schaeffer's group proved irrefutably that the cytoplasm of a tumor cell could initiate and drive cancer, it was impossible to ignore the results. Schaeffer claimed, "Here we present the data which, for the first time, provide unambiguous evidence indicating a role for cytoplasm in the expression of the malignant phenotype." Rather than shaking the foundation of cancer biology, the claim was ignored—even worse than being argued against.

The beautiful experiments were loaded with theoretical implications, and some would argue that they should have altered the trajectory of a portion of NCI money. But NCI made the decision that the experiments, with their astonishing connotations, merited no further exploration. If Seyfried had not dug them up, they may well have been forgotten. Seyfried reflected on the lost importance of the experiments, saying, "In summary, the origin of carcinogenesis resides with the mitochondria in the cytoplasm, not with the genome in the nucleus."

How was it possible that so many in the cancer field seemed unaware of the evidence supporting this concept? How could so many ignore the findings while embracing the gene theory? Perhaps Rous was correct when he said "the SMT acts like a tranquilizer on those who believe in it." The results of these carefully conducted and duplicated experiments seemed inescapable: cancer was driven by the cytoplasm, as Warburg claimed.

Schaeffer said,

My only thoughts then, as now, is that the results we obtained were due to epigenetic effects. Obviously, since the nuclei were obtained, free of cytoplasm and were then fused into cells from which the nucleus was removed, one also has to take into consideration the effect of mitochondria. Something akin to nuclear/

cytoplasmic incompatibility. That was also the thinking of Junichi Hyashi, then a postdoc with Jerry Shay in Texas. We talked about this a great deal. Unfortunately, the wisdom (or lack of it) from NIH study committees would not entertain such an idea at the time.

Schaeffer felt the experiments deserved more attention and funding, but NIH was focused on genetics and was not about to change course.

Instinctually Schaeffer felt the experiments revealed an important clue into the fundamental nature of cancer, but he was frustrated that NCI was happy to ignore the results. He revealed another reason why the results may have been lost into a vacuum: "I have to admit that what confounded us in our work was that we, too, were stuck on the genetic origin. How to reconcile our findings with that theory?" After he learned more about the reemerging metabolic theory of cancer, he couldn't help but to nostalgically reflect on the irony of his career:

Also, at that time, I was not aware of the metabolic research even though I was familiar with Warburg (I spent the greater part of my PhD research work using the Warburg apparatus). However, putting that together with our work should have caused us, in retrospect, to delve further into the earliest research involving mitochondria. Where was Seyfried when we could have used him????

As far as Jerry Shay, he seemed to have moved on to other pursuits. While Shay and Schaeffer were performing the experiments, they had no theoretical framework from which to extrapolate the meaning of the results. Seyfried's version of the metabolic theory of cancer didn't exist, Warburg was forgotten, and Pedersen was working in isolation. Seyfried said, "The beauty of it is that none of these people were doing these experiments specifically to test the (Warburg) hypothesis. It was tested unknowingly by the person doing the experiment, so you couldn't ask for anything less biased."

Things May Not Be as They Seem

In 2003, after the hype surrounding Herceptin had faded, a new drug, imatinib, stole the spotlight. The new drug was brand named GLEEVEC, and like Herceptin, it targeted a specific mutation. This one was found in a rare subset of leukemia called chronic myeloid leukemia (CML), a disease that tended to strike people in middle age. Unlike Herceptin's tepid results, GLEEVEC'S results were remarkable. It was the first targeted cancer drug synonymous with the word "cure."

In 2000, one year before GLEEVEC was approved by the FDA, 2,300 people died from CML. By 2009, that number had fallen to 470, all due to GLEEVEC. Though the results equated to only a fraction of lives in the overall war, less than one-third of 1 percent each year, they did not go unnoticed. The cover of *Time* displayed a picture of the orange pills and the caption, "There Is New Ammunition in the War against Cancer—These Are the Bullets." Perhaps more than the drug itself, GLEEVEC represented a much-needed symbol of victory, a sign that researchers were pursuing the right concept with regard to drug design. It served to "justify an approach," as one researcher put it. As if erupting from decades of pent-up frustration, the hyperbole exploded into the media. GLEEVEC was described by an experienced cancer researcher in the *New York Times* as "the beginning of a sea change—and I am speaking conservatively—in the way we practice cancer medicine."

Varmus weighed in on the subject in an essay titled "The New Era in Cancer Research." Perhaps more than anyone, he was responsible for drawing the blueprint used for drug design, and he must have felt vindicated on some level. Brian Druker, the MD who helped refine the drug in its infancy and fought to get GLEEVEC pushed through the clinic, wrote that GLEEVEC was a "paradigm shift in cancer drug development." The phrase most often showered on the drug was "proof of principle," proving that the scientific foundation built by the SMT of cancer was the right starting point when designing any therapy. The story of GLEEVEC was not one of a victory in the war against cancer but one of vindication, proving that researchers weren't struggling in vain.

The story of GLEEVEC began in 1960 when a physician named Peter Nowell and a graduate student, thrust into a small lab in Philadelphia, looked at a slide covered with cells from a CML patient. They noticed something odd. One of the chromosomes in the CML cells appeared shorter compared to its partner, but they weren't sure, because the difference was minute. So they retrieved CML cells from a different patient and looked again. Again they saw the shortened chromosome, like a midget standing next to its taller twin. They got samples from five more patients, and all had the same shortened chromosome. They thought that perhaps it was a genetic anomaly general to all types of leukemia, so they looked at the chromosomes of other forms of leukemia. This time the dwarf chromosome wasn't to be found, it appeared that the anomaly was specific to CML.

In 1960, they published the findings, suggesting a causal link between the genetic anomaly and CML. But without the techniques to derive the significance of Nowell's discovery, it was left as a curious observation, and it was twelve years before the strange genetic lesion was revisited.

An MD in Chicago named Janet Rowley, armed with a new chromosomal staining technique, looked at the shortened chromosome and was able to sort out the details. The shortened chromosome that

Nowell had observed had a chunk that was lopped off and stitched onto a different chromosome. The transfer was from chromosome 22 to chromosome 9. When Rowley looked closer, she noticed that it wasn't a transfer but rather a swap—chromosome 9 had also transferred a smaller piece to chromosome 22. By itself, the swap was meaningless, but the product of the new genetic material had meaning.

The protein product of the altered genetic material acted out the malevolent effects of the unnatural union. The swap of the Abelson (abl) tyrosine kinase gene at chromosome 9 and break point cluster (Bcr) gene at chromosome 22 resulted in the chimerical oncogene Bcr-abl. The product of this hybrid was a Frankenstein-like kinase. Like src, it was an overactive tyrosine kinase, a signal molecule with its switch stuck in the "on" position. It was nicknamed "the Philadelphia chromosome," because that was where Nowell discovered it, and with the specific molecular details worked out, now the question was whether it could be stopped.

The story of GLEEVEC moved across the Atlantic to Switzerland where a chemist named Jurg Zimmermann was working with a class of molecules called phenylamine-pyrimidines (PAPs) at the pharmaceutical company Ciba-Geigy. Zimmermann was tipped off by a professor from a nearby university that certain PAPs might inhibit kinases, the proteins often vilified as the cause of cancer. Targeting a kinase was thought to be impossible. They were too structurally similar to each other, and there was too many of them. A drug would have to be remarkably specific, or it would probably inhibit a host of other kinases, which would be extremely detrimental to the cell.

But Zimmermann was undeterred. The process was trial and error on a massive scale, like randomly cutting multitudes of keys to see which one fit a lock. Zimmerman plowed through the tedious process and eventually developed a short list of compounds that proved adept at inhibiting certain kinases. It wasn't long before he tried them on

Bcr-abl. When he ran the experiments, some of the PAPs proved skillful at inhibiting or turning Bcr-abl "off." A drug specific to Bcr-abl was tantalizing, but it would have to be optimized. The drug would have to exhibit laser-like specificity.

The significance of the discovery was not lost on Nicholas Lydon, the head of Zimmerman's development team. He understood that Bcr-abl alone was responsible for CML, and to inhibit it meant possibly curing this simple form of cancer. Before they got the chance to fine-tune the details, they encountered an obstacle.

In 1996, Ciba-Geigy announced that it was merging with another Swiss company, Sandoz, to form the pharmaceutical juggernaut Novartis. In the wake of mergers, companies typically try to slough off departments judged to be redundant, and Novartis was no different. Lydon's group was considered low priority. Like the Slamon-Ullrich relationship supplied the technical punch necessary for Genentech to take a risk on Herceptin, Lydon met the man who would help him save the program and move it to the top of the list. Armed with a freezer full of potential candidates to slip in the mutated pocket of the Bcr-abl kinase, Lydon needed sensitive tests determine which one worked best.

He traveled to the Dana Farber Cancer Institute in Boston where exquisite tests had been developed to test kinase inhibitors. In Boston, Lydon met Brian Druker, a young faculty member who shared an intense interest in Bcr-abl. Druker also had access to something else Lydon needed: patients. They plotted an ambitious partnership. They would isolate the best candidate and then try it on CMT patients, but they had difficulty convincing the top brass at Novartis that the idea was worth the investment. The accountants had legitimate concerns. It could cost up to $100 million to move a drug through the clinic with no guarantee of success. In addition, because of the targeted nature of the drug, it had only a tiny market to serve, making return on investment difficult. Druker refused to give up, and in the end, his passion overwhelmed everyone's reservations.

The first man to receive GLEEVEC was a sixty-year-old retired train conductor from the Oregon coast. Like Ko a decade later, Druker sat nervously by the bed while the drug was administered. The same overwhelming sense of relief that would break Ko into tears struck Druker once it was apparent that GLEEVEC wasn't acutely toxic. "The sense of relief was incredible," Druker said, but something even more incredible was to come.

The first trial included fifty-four patients, and fifty-three exhibited a complete response within days of starting the drug. As enough time passed, it became apparent that GLEEVEC was able to keep the cancer at bay—it never returned. The results reverberated through the cancer research community and then the world at large. Because of GLEEVEC, a disease that was once fatal three to five years after diagnosis could be managed, and the patient usually lived a normal lifespan.

Perhaps no other cancer therapy had such a profound impact on the institution of oncology than GLEEVEC. So much so, its symbolic power cut a line through cancer's history; doctors now often reference a "pre-GLEEVEC era" and a "post-GLEEVEC era." Oncologists had waited desperately for GLEEVEC, they finally had a nontoxic cure in their tool kit. They could look a patient in the eye and say, "It is going to be okay."

GLEEVEC is a dream child, the holy grail of chemotherapy: a non-toxic cure. But GLEEVEC carries a hidden danger. Beyond its other-worldly impact, it solidified the logic of targeted cancer therapy. It alone "justified an approach" or served as "proof of principle," again locking researchers into a myopic vision of drug design. The problem lay with the fact that as far as cancers go, CML is unique. Unlike the vast majority of the solid tumors, CML is remarkably homogeneous.

While most solid tumors display a hurricane of genetic chaos, CML is pure, its genetic landscape dominated by a single alteration: the Philadelphia chromosome. Author Clifton Leaf put it this way, "The danger of the targeted drug revolution—of The GLEEVEC Story—is that it oversimplified cancer, treating the disease as an orderly march to disorder, the result of a lone, driving genetic aberration. That is not the case with the vast majority of cancers."

GLEEVEC directed researchers down a perilous path even when operating within the framework of genetics. The vast majority of cancers are too complex to apply the "GLEEVEC model" to them. Watson admitted that it might be an impossible task, as did Loeb, as did Vogelstein.

GLEEVEC carries another danger. Beyond serving as a proof of principle for targeted drug design, GLEEVEC seems to validate the SMT of cancer on the surface. It appears that CMT originates and progresses due to a single, pervasive genetic alteration. Digging deeper, researchers found that the Philadelphia chromosome *exists in perfectly healthy people who will never develop CML*—this was a small but critical detail. *That simply cannot be.* If the Philadelphia chromosome alone caused CMT, these blissfully ignorant individuals should harbor the malignancy, but this is not the case. The out-of-control kinase produced by Bcr-abl is not enough by itself to cause CML. Further, more advanced cases of CML are not always treatable by GLEEVEC. Twenty percent of advanced cases succumb to CML even with GLEEVEC and even with a single supposed "founding" mutation that permeates the entire genetic landscape of the cancer—a single mutation that a targeted therapy could grab hold of in every cancer cell, not just a fraction. These two facts provide clear proof that something else beyond Bcr-abl is driving the disease.

Pedersen and Seyfried have noticed something else curious about GLEEVEC. They noticed that the *how* of GLEEVEC inconspicuously converges with the metabolic theory. The wildly hyperactive kinase Bcr-abl leads to the permanent activation of a network called the PI3K/AKT pathway. The pathway is also activated by damaged mitochondria followed by the retrograde response. Whether the pathway is activated by the retrograde response or by Bcr-abl, a quiver of specific genes are aroused from their slumber, and cajoled to order the manufacture of a network of proteins that then manipulate the biochemical personality of the cell toward the Warburg effect with all its manifestations. The PI3K/AKT pathway dramatically increases glucose uptake and use. When CML patients swallow an orange GLEEVEC pill, their cancer cells lose their insatiable appetite for glucose, and oxidative energy creation is restored, a reversal of the Warburg effect. It should raise eyebrows that the one targeted drug out of seven hundred, the drug that was a home run, exerts it effect by shutting down Warburg's metabolic pathway. Coincidences are not evidence by themselves, but neither do they exist in a vacuum. One that spun out of a one-in-seven-hundred chance should command some respect.

Additionally, Ko and Pedersen ran experiments comparing the activity of 3BP and GLEEVEC in multiple myeloma cells, a cancer without the Philadelphia chromosome. While 3BP was better than GLEEVEC in combating the cells, Ko and Pedersen couldn't help but notice that GLEEVEC appeared to exert its anticancer effect by depleting cellular ATP. This was a curious observation for a drug recognized for its exquisite specificity. Ko said,

It is worth noting that GLEEVEC kills RPM18226 cancer cells by depleting cellular ATP. Therefore, it is speculated that GLEEVEC acts as a metabolic inhibitor by binding nonspecifically to several tyrosine kinases and ATP binding/hydrolyzing proteins including ATP synthomes. Significantly, our results are consistent with the view of Dr. Thomas Seyfried that cancer is a disease of energy metabolism.

The GLEEVEC paradigm has provided a collective sense of relief to the cancer community. As intellectually satisfying as GLEEVEC is, below the surface it is anything but. When all the facts are taken together, even the elegant simplicity of GLEEVEC is shrouded in a veil of contradiction. It could be that CML has a strong, purely genetic component driven by a kinase gone mad. Or, it could be that Bcr-abl is just a serendipitous switch, rather than the cause of CML. It is just a means to an end, a tool, used to turn off the signal turned on by damaged mitochondria.

Seyfried pointed out another line of evidence that, when examined closely, appears to be a wash. Historically, inherited mutations were often cited as evidence supporting the SMT of cancer, and on the surface, this appears to be true. Germline (passed from parent to offspring) mutations that resulted in cancer account for a small part of the overall burden (5–7 percent of all cancers). The overwhelming majority of cancers arise spontaneously. There could be no doubt that certain germline mutations predispose afflicted individuals to developing cancer, but as with carcinogens and GLEEVEC, it is the *how* that again blurs the distinction between the competing theories.

The protein products of oncogenes are anything but simple. They display an incredibly complex and diverse functionality. P53, the most studied oncogene, has conservatively been shown to interact with 105 other proteins, combining to affect an incomprehensibly vast network of cellular operations. P53 is biblical in nature, and like the Bible, its importance depends on the interpreter. Proponents of the SMT see p53 as the "guardian of the genome"—its mission is to protect the kingdom. When the nuclear walls are breached, p53 orchestrates legions of workers to repair any damage. If the damage is too extensive to be repaired, p53 sounds the trumpets, ordering the cell to commit suicide before it can be corrupted.

Proponents of the metabolic theory see p53's mission as crucial to maintaining oxidative energy generation. P53 is responsible for the transcription of a critical component of the electron transport chain without which the mitochondria can't do its job. Persons born with a germline mutation to p53 have an almost certain chance of developing cancer in their lifetime, and 50 percent of people with the rare disorder develop tumors in early adulthood. (The condition is called Li-Fraumeni syndrome.) The question is *how* the inherited p53 mutation is causing the increased predisposition to cancer. Most cancer biologists say that it is because the genome is left vulnerable, increasing the chances that a mutation will strike other critical proto-oncogenes. Proponents of the metabolic theory say that mutated p53 slowly erodes the cell's ability to generate energy oxidatively. This results in a conversion to the Warburg effect followed by the retrograde response and uncontrolled growth.

The same holds true with BRCA1; this inherited mutation conveys a much greater chance that afflicted women will develop breast and ovarian cancer. BRCA1 received a burst of media attention when the actress Angelina Jolie announced her decision to undergo a double mastectomy in a 2013 *New York Times* op-ed titled "My Medical Choice." After she tested positive for the BRCA1 gene, she decided to undergo the procedure. Doctors estimated that she had an 87 percent chance of developing breast cancer, and her procedure reduced her chances to 5 percent. It was likely that she inherited the faulty gene from her mother, who died of breast cancer at age fifty-six. "Once I knew that this was my reality, I decided to be proactive and to minimize the risk as much I could," Jolie wrote. She went public with her decision to inform others who might be at risk so that they could be proactive and their fate need not be sealed in Darwinian inevitability. She wrote,

I choose not to keep my story private, because there are many women who do not know that they might be living under the shadow of cancer. It is my hope that they, too, will be able to get gene tested, and that if they have a high risk they, too, will know that they have strong options. Life comes with many challenges. The ones that should not scare us are the ones we can take on and take control of.

Like p53, BRCA1 has multiple cellular functions, and also like p53, the BRCA1 protein is one of the many proteins responsible for the repair of DNA damage. BRCA1 does not cause cancer directly, rather, proponents of the SMT contend that it allows it to happen. It sets the stage. It increases the *likelihood* of mutations that unhinged proliferation. And like p53, it is also implicated in mitochondrial function. It has been shown to be intimately involved in the biogenesis of mitochondria. The faulty version could limit the mitochondria's ability to reproduce, leading to the tremendously reduced numbers within the cytoplasm of cancer cells that Pedersen and others have seen.

The same dual nature holds true for other inherited mutations that increase the risk of developing cancer. These included retinoblastoma, xeroderma pigmentosum, paraganglioma, and some forms of renal cell carcinoma. All the inherited mutations implicated have been shown to impair mitochondrial function – a critical detail that is still largely ignored.

Superfuel

Starting with the observation that cancer was tied to metabolism, Seyfried began a pilgrimage to understand why. The broad circle he began with arced into a tighter trajectory, forming smaller circles until he arrived at the center: a single metabolic theory of cancer.

Mitochondria: An Old Theory Is New Again

Like a star collapsing in on itself, his work exploded outward to the therapeutic question with which it began. With a comprehensive theory in place and a framework of understanding built, his lab could use the theory as a starting point and a filter to design therapies to treat cancer.

Seyfried noticed that simple caloric restriction shrank tumors, an observation that he could now extrapolate through a theoretical framework. Now it made sense. Caloric restriction drives down blood glucose, forcing cancer cells to ferociously compete with healthy cells for the fuel they so desperately crave. But he reasoned he might be able to do better. He modified the diet slightly, keeping overall calories restricted but eliminating carbohydrates in favor of fats, a modification that might put even more metabolic pressure on the cancer cells. With no carbohydrates, the body is jerked out of its normal state of metabolic energy generation. It is forced to manufacture molecules called ketone bodies to take the place of glucose as a source of circulating fuel. Once cancer is framed as a metabolic disease, ketone bodies have an interesting therapeutic potential.

Unlike glucose, ketone bodies burn oxidatively. They have to be burned in healthy, functioning mitochondria, something that Seyfried knew cancer cells don't have many of. Metabolically, normal cells have other options, but cancer cells do not. If cancer was truly a disease of dysfunctional mitochondria, a dietary regimen that he coined the "restricted ketogenic diet" (R-KD), one that transitions away from glucose to ketone bodies, might have more impact than simple caloric restriction.

His line of reasoning extended back to ancient Greece when the therapeutic value of fasting was discovered. It was noticed that fasting markedly reduced, if not completely stopped, epileptic seizures. In the 1920s, around the time that Warburg was documenting the striking metabolic differences in cancer cells, Rollin Woodyatt, a physician scientist in Chicago, reported that three water-soluble ketone bodies (B-hydroxybutyrate, acetoacetate, and acetone) were manufactured by the liver in healthy people who were fasting or eating a diet low in carbohydrate and high in fat.

Inspired by the metabolic shift that Woodyatt observed, a Mayo Clinic physician named Russell Wilder developed a diet that mimicked fasting by producing ketone bodies but could be maintained indefinitely. He reasoned that the diet could be used therapeutically for victims of epilepsy. Wilder's diet, which he termed the ketogenic diet, consisted of approximately one gram of protein per kilogram of body weight per day with almost no carbohydrates and the rest of the calories from fat. The results for those with epilepsy were profound. The ketogenic diet significantly reduced the number of seizures or eliminated them altogether. However, when anticonvulsive medications were developed in the 1940s, the ketogenic diet was relegated to a sidenote in medical textbooks.

In the mid-1990s, the diet was pulled from obscurity and thrust into the limelight by Hollywood movie director Jim Abrahams. His son, Charlie, had a severe form of epilepsy that refused to respond to medication. Charlie's life was hijacked by the frequency and severity of the seizures. "It was a fate worse than death," Abrahams said. After visiting five neurologists who had no answers, he was desperate to try anything. "Once I heard about the ketogenic diet, we tried it—within days Charlie was seizure free. I was baffled and angry at the time. How could the public not know about this?" he said.

He set off on a crusade to inform others who might be in the same desperate situation. He appeared on NBC's *Dateline* and produced a made-for-TV movie titled *First Do No Harm* starring his good friend Meryl Streep. He then started the Charlie Foundation dedicated to training dieticians in hospitals to administer the ketogenic diet for epileptics, but his efforts encountered friction.

Mitochondria: An Old Theory Is New Again

When I started the Charlie Foundation, I thought it would be a straight line—we would inform the public of this incredibly effective dietary treatment for epilepsy, and that would be it. Unfortunately, it wasn't that simple. Today all the myths that had been used to detract from the diet have been disproven. Efficacy had been scientifically established, fears of negative effects from long term use have been dispelled, palatability has been dramatically enhanced, and difficulty of administration has been equally dramatically reduced. The biggest problem today is trying to figure out how hospitals can reimburse trained ketogenic diet dietitians for their time.

Richard Veech at NIH knows the science behind the ketogenic diet perhaps better than anyone. Fittingly, he is also a member of the scientific lineage leading directly back to Warburg. He received his PhD under Hans Krebs at Oxford (who studied under Warburg and, after Warburg's death, wrote his biography). Veech, among others, noticed the almost magical properties of ketone bodies. He was intrigued by a report from 1940s showing that ketone bodies were unique among sixteen other carbohydrates, fatty acids, and intermediate metabolites in their ability to increase the mobility of sperm while decreasing the amount of oxygen consumed. Ketone bodies turned them into faster, more efficient swimmers. Determined to see if the study was true, Veech added ketone bodies to a glucose solution containing rat heart muscle. The ketone bodies increased the amount of work performed by the heart muscle while significantly decreasing oxygen consumption. Veech then noticed something else. Not only did the ketone bodies result in greater efficiency, but they showed a strange ability to drastically increase the amount of ATP produced inside the cell. He discovered that by widening a critical energetic gap in the electron transport chain, ketone bodies changed the intracellular landscape, supercharging the cell. The metabolic transformation inspired him to dub the molecules "superfuel."

He then took a bird's-eye view of the obscure fuel and attempted to figure out how ketone bodies came to exist in the first place. He concluded that the molecules probably helped our ancestors develop a larger, more complex brain. In terms of survival advantage, the larger brain gave us a leg up on every other species, but in strictly metabolic terms, it was an enormous burden—it had an insatiable appetite. The brain consumes 20 percent of the energy from food at any given time. Worse, while other tissues in the body can transition to burning fatty acids, the brain is hamstrung by the fact it can only burn glucose, leaving it uniquely vulnerable. When food was a scarce resource—as no doubt frequently occurred—our best friend turned into our worst enemy. But evolution found a solution: a metabolic conversion during times of deprivation into a state of hyper efficiency or ketosis. Because the brain could transition from burning glucose to ketone bodies, the molecules could rescue the brain from its metabolic intransigence, providing a back-up fuel to feed its monstrous appetite. Humans more than any other mammal can produce "superfuel" in lean times, making us gritty, efficient survival machines.

Veech said, "The survival benefit is obvious; ketone bodies allow a normal-weight human to go from two to three weeks without food to about two months. An obese man can live close to a year without food." From an evolutionary standpoint, it may be impossible to separate the two: ketosis may have facilitated or allowed our huge brains to evolve in the first place.

Ketone bodies made sense when viewed as an evolutionary adaptation, but how they worked to stop epileptic seizures, as in Charlie's case, is still a mystery. Veech's work led to renewed interest in the physiological effects of ketone bodies, inspiring other researchers to investigate the mysterious molecules, and the results were almost too good to believe.

In addition to the well-known weight-loss benefits that Robert Atkins kicked off in the 1970s, ketosis was shown to potentially impact a host of neurological diseases including Parkinson's disease, Alzheimer's disease, ALS, and brain trauma. The seemingly magical properties of ketone bodies flew in the face of Veech's scientific skepticism. He said, "These diseases appear wildly different," and treating "all these different things with some magic substance sounds improbable." But the molecules, time after time, showed a broad neuroprotective effect. The benefits from ketosis circled back to the mitochondria. Because ketone bodies are used so efficiently, they reduce the oxidative burden imposed on mitochondria from energy creation. Like a cleaner-burning fuel, ketone bodies appear to preserve, or even restore, damaged mitochondria. But, viewed from another angle the almost miraculous effects of ketone bodies may not be so miraculous after all. Maybe humans were supposed to exist in the state of ketosis from time to time. As Veech said in an article in the *New York Times*, "Ketosis is a normal physiological state. I would argue it is the normal state of man. It's not normal to have a McDonald's and a delicatessen around every corner. It's normal to starve." Maybe many modern diseases were an artifact of civilization, and maybe, as Veech suggested, a little deprivation did us a ton of good.

Starting with the idea that cancer needs glucose and that cancer cells have drastically reduced numbers of mitochondria, damaged mitochondria, or both, Seyfried modified the ketogenic diet to put as much metabolic stress on the cancer cell as possible. He restricted the overall calories in order to drive blood glucose down as far as possible, depriving the cancer cells of their preferred fuel. Healthy cells will transition to burning ketone bodies in their intact mitochondria, something that cancer cells are unable to do. Seyfried found that this restricted version of the ketogenic diet dramatically slowed the growth of tumors in mice.

The idea that restricting calories effects tumor growth circled back to Rous. In 1914, Rous wondered if diet could influence the vascularity of tumors; the expanding network of vessels that allowed tumors to grow and infiltrate. In a paper titled "The Influence of Diet on Transplanted and Spontaneous Mouse Tumors," Rous provided striking evidence that a restriction in food intake starved the ability of tumors to grow. Rous said, "In these facts may be found the method whereby dieting delays tumor growth. With a lessened proliferative activity of the host tissue, the elaboration of a vascularizing and supporting stroma such as most tumors depend upon for their growth, at least indirectly, is much delayed." Because his finding came before Warburg, the idea had nothing to anchor to, and his observation remained a free-floating anomaly.

Warburg made a loose dietary connection to cancer from a different angle:

To prevent cancer, it is therefore proposed first to keep the speed of the blood stream so high that the venous blood still contains sufficient oxygen; second, to keep high the concentration of hemoglobin in the blood; third, to add always to the food, even of healthy people, the active groups of the respiratory enzymes; and to increase the doses of these groups, if a precancerous state has already developed. If at the same time exogenous carcinogens are excluded rigorously, then much of the endogenous cancer may be prevented today. These proposals are in no way utopian. On the contrary, they may be realized by everybody, everywhere, at any hour. Unlike the prevention of many other diseases, the prevention of cancer requires no government help, and not much money.

Mitochondria: An Old Theory Is New Again

Like many before and after him, he suggested that the best way to chip away at the cancer burden was through prevention. His ideas focused on maintaining the fidelity of the respiratory apparatus through exercise, respiratory vitamins (mostly B vitamins), and the avoidance of carcinogens (a practice that Warburg took to an extreme; in his later years, he ate only food grown organically on his own land).

The first documented use of the ketogenic diet in cancer came in 1995 by Linda Nebeling. Nebeling found her way into nutrition more by default than design. Unsure if she wanted to be a veterinarian or a medical doctor, she decided to get an undergraduate degree in nutrition and leave both options open. After graduating, having family in New York, she applied for a nutritionist internship at Sloan Kettering Hospital. She was captivated by the "groundbreaking" nutritional protocols implemented there. She found the transition from the sleepy halls of academia to the fast-paced atmosphere at Sloan Kettering Hospital intoxicating. "The AIDS epidemic was hitting the area hard," Nebeling said. "It was a challenging time as a nutritionist."

But she found herself more drawn to the cancer ward than the challenges presented by the strange new virus. Cancer can present many challenges for a nutritionist, especially the problem of cachexia, a wasting syndrome that tends to strike cancer patients in the late throes of the disease. The chronic condition can not be easily reversed by nutrition. She began to think about the nutritional side of cancer from a different angle. Perhaps nutrition could be used to attenuate the side effects or even alter the course of certain types of cancer. Full of inspiration and charged with creativity, she wanted to be in an experimental environment that allowed her to explore the boundaries of nutrition, and that meant returning to academia. She left New York to begin her PhD work at Case Western Reserve in Ohio.

In the new environment she began to formulate a question: could cancer be altered by diet alone? Her question led to a series of discussions with an oncologist who shared her interest, and they eventually arrived at the ketogenic diet. "I knew the diet was effective against seizures in pediatric epilepsy, and so it had some effect neurologically," Nebeling said. She made the connection between the tumor's reliance on glucose and the diet's shift away from glucose. Her ideas were perfectly timed. PET scanning was gaining ground as a valuable diagnostic procedure, and it had made its way into the clinic where she worked. It was a perfect collision of theory and technology. Nebeling realized that it would allow her to see if the diet was having an effect. "It was a blending of nutrition with pediatric oncology with PET scanning," she said.

It took a year for her to get the procedure in place. Once the approvals were ready, she just needed patients. "I screened over twenty-five before I found two who would fit the protocol." The first patient was a three-year-old girl diagnosed with stage 4 anaplastic astrocytoma. Before entering Nebeling's trial, the child had received the "eight drugs in one day" regimen. This involved the administration of highly toxic drugs with steroids followed by hyperfractionated radiation therapy to the head and spine. The child experienced seizures and suffered from extensive blood and renal toxicity. Her treatment was halted due to continued tumor progression.

The second patient was a girl, eight and a half years old, diagnosed with grade 3 cerebellar astrocytoma—it had progressed from a low-grade tumor diagnosed at age six. The girl suffered hearing loss from cisplatin toxicity.

Both patients still had measurable tumors after extensive treatment and both had the same grim prognosis. After failing treatment, neither girl was expected to live more than three years.

Over the course of a week, Nebeling transitioned the girls to the mildly restrictive ketogenic diet. Both girls had family willing to help, so Nebeling taught the families how to follow the diet. By periodically measuring ketones, she was able to tell if the families were complying with the strict diet. Although "adherence to the diet was not perfect," Nebeling said, for the most part they stayed true to course. "Consumption of the diet was not a major limitation for the patients, but if we could have developed a ketosis-compliant Oreo cookie, it would have been a big hit," Nebeling said. Even though the girls maintained their body weight, their blood glucose dropped to below normal while their blood ketones increased twenty or thirty fold. As time passed, the seizures one girl experienced prior to the diet stopped, and her overall quality of life began to improve.

As encouraging as the results appeared, PET scans would show if the diet was choking off the sweet tooth of the tumors. When Nebeling received the results, they revealed a 22 percent reduction in uptake, reflecting a sharp decrease in glucose consumption. Over the nine-month course of the protocol, Nebeling meticulously monitored the girls, adjusting their diet if they got a cold and performing blood tests to ensure that they were properly nourished.

Though the study was not designed to measure outcome, Nebeling admitted to the diet's seductive potential to starve cancer cells of their dependence on glucose. She said, "Theoretically, the effect on the rate of glucose use at the tumor site may impact the rate of tumor growth." But she was quick to snap back into the original mission: "That said, the protocol was not designed to reverse tumor growth or treat specific types of cancer." Even if the protocol was never designed to "treat" the girls, the families had pinned their hopes on the diet. How could they not? The PET scan results suggested it was having an effect—the three-year-old girl had recovered from the gut-wrenching side effects of conventional chemotherapy and radiation, and both girls were feeling better.

A year passed, and Nebeling had enough data from the trial to complete her PhD. She transitioned from hands-on dietician to academic as she summarized the data for her dissertation. She applied for a post-doc fellowship at NCI, hoping to continue her focus on cancer. When she heard that she had been selected for the fellowship, she was elated but a little sad, because it meant that she would have to leave the girls. "They were in good hands at the University Hospitals of Cleveland," she said. She packed her bags and moved to Washington, DC.

Nebeling's theoretically elegant idea that cancer's defective metabolism could be exploited through diet had slowly worked its way into the imaginations of scientists and the public. In the summer of 2007, *Time* ran an article titled "Can a High-Fat Diet Beat Cancer?" It focused on two German scientists, Dr. Melanie Schmidt and biologist Ulrike Kämmerer who began a phase 1 trial at the famous University Hospital of Wurzburg to test the ketogenic diet in cancer patients. Underwritten by the German food company Tavartis, the experiment expanded on Nebeling's trial and was designed to see if the diet could have an impact on the course of the disease. In the article, the scientists were quoted as saying "Whether Warburg was right or not is irrelevant." They believed that their famous countryman had identified a target that they hoped to exploit. Even though they were allowed to recruit only extremely ill patients who had run out of any therapeutic options, they saw positive results.

Nebeling's results were also mentioned in the article. When the article was published, Nebeling had lost contact with both girls, but through colleagues at the University Hospitals of Cleveland, she confirmed in 2005 that the younger patient was alive and doing well—fifteen years after the girl had been told that there was nothing left to do and that she probably had three years left to live.

Even though Nebeling was quick to point out that the pilot study was too small to draw any definitive conclusions, the results were conspicuous. Both girls weren't expected to live more than three years from the time they started the ketogenic diet, but one had lived at least ten years and the other at least fifteen years beyond the prognosis.

The short Wurzburg trial confirmed what Nebeling's study alluded to: the diet seemed to be affecting the growth of cancer cells. Of the five patients who completed the three-month trial, all remained alive, with their tumor's growth either slowing, stopping, or, in some cases, shrinking.

Nemesis

In 2000, Seyfried's stumble into the metabolism of cancer was for the most part triggered by one question: why would caloric restriction slow the growth of cancer? The question spiraled into a head-first immersion into the biochemical guts of the cancer cell. He found that below the surface both caloric restriction and R-KD were affecting a vast swath of biochemical processes. He found that mirroring the ability of ketone bodies to attenuate a host of seemingly unrelated neurological diseases, caloric restriction effected many qualitative aspects of the cancer cell. As before, the findings appeared too good to be true.

He found the R-KD to be *antiangiogenic*—it choked off the production of new blood vessels supplying the tumor, as Rous discovered almost one hundred years earlier. The diet was also *proapoptotic*, in that it facilitated orderly cell death. This was in sharp contrast to the chaotic cell death of chemotherapy and radiation, a disorderly process known to increase inflammation and fan the flames of malignancy. As practitioners of periodic fasting or caloric restriction had documented for years, the diet proved to be anti-inflammatory, a loosely defined process associated with initiating and driving cancer.

Seyfried looked further, the diet proved to be anti-invasive. Very aggressive mouse models of metastatic cancer spread to fewer sites while on the diet. The diet influenced hormones like IGF-1, implicated as fuel for tumor cells, attenuating its malevolent influence. It turned down the PI3K/AKT pathway, the same pathway that GLEEVEC was found to influence. Everywhere he looked, every biochemical process subverted by cancer, the diet pushed back, pressuring the cells to a state of normality. "All oncologists should know that dietary restriction is the nemesis of many cancers," he wrote in his book.

Sifting the data through Seyfried's metabolic theory of cancer and bending the restricted diet toward a high-fat ketogenic diet made mechanistic and strategic sense, especially in light of Nebeling's results. Other researchers did experiments that added weight to the idea. One experiment added ketone bodies to a petri dish containing growing cancer cells and one containing normal cells. As suspected, the cancer cells died or floundered along, barely able to grow, while the normal cells effortlessly transitioned to the new fuel. The evidence pointing to the logic of the approach bombarded Seyfried from every angle.

By 2008, Seyfried felt that he had enough evidence to try the restricted version of the ketogenic diet in a human patient. In choosing a type of cancer, he tried to stack the likelihood of achieving positive results in his favor. Brain cancer was the best candidate, because the brain was 100 percent reliant on glucose for fuel, but it could also seamlessly transition to ketone body metabolism. It's unique "one or the other" metabolism seemed ideally suited for the regime.

Just before Christmas of 2008, Dr. Giulio Zuccoli was informed that his sister had found their mother, Marianne, confused and praying in church—she couldn't remember why she had decided to enter the church, how she had gotten there, or what she was praying about. When Zuccoli heard the story, he suspected that it was the same thing his father had died from a year earlier. She had been having chronic headaches and nausea. All of the symptoms combined, along with her "seizure-like" episode at the church – the same symptoms his father had gone through—consolidated the diagnosis in his mind.

Mitochondria: An Old Theory Is New Again

An MRI revealed that his instincts were right. Marianne had glioblastoma, the most dreaded form of brain cancer. The scans revealed a large, multicentric mass that had infiltrating tentacles in almost every direction. It would be impossible to fully remove it. Zuccoli knew that the diagnosis carried a fixed outcome, and his beloved mother was going to die. Knowing full well that the standard of care offered no hope of survival, Zuccoli and his mother decided to complement it with an alternative approach: a dietary regimen based on the work of Seyfried at Boston College. Although Zuccoli's colleagues questioned his decision, the metabolic approach made sense to him. Over a series of conversations, he and Seyfried determined a course of action. They would put Marianne on R-KD alongside the normal standard of care, radiation and chemotherapy.

The debulking surgery went as well as expected. As much of the malignancy was removed as possible, but portions of the matrix-like mass eluded them. On December 16, six days after surgery, Marianne felt up to initiating the diet. Zuccoli explained to her the logic behind the dietary trial. Cancer needed sugar to grow, so the diet removed as much sugar as possible. He told her that if she felt up to it, fasting would be the best way to begin. Still in the intensive care unit, she began a water-only fast. Her son held her hand, gently supporting her.

After twenty-four hours, she shifted to a low-calorie diet. After five days on the low-calorie diet, they again initiated a water-only fast, this time maintaining it for three days. At the end of the third day, the dietician put her on R-KD. It consisted of 600 calories a day of mostly fat and some protein, removing any food that could be easily converted into sugar. Her blood sugar plummeted from 120 to 60, and her ketones shot through the roof. On January 8, she started radiation and chemotherapy.

Seyfried convinced Zuccoli to hold off on the typical steroid medication designed to combat the tissue damage caused by radiation. It could dramatically raise blood glucose levels and negate what they were attempting to do with the diet. The radiation and chemo were stopped on February 17.

The first MRI was a week later. Marianne wasn't nervous about the results, but "she was simply contemplative," Zuccoli said. He read her the results: "No evidence of any tumor." The difference between the MRI taken the day she entered the hospital and the one just taken was striking. Where there were once grotesque masses, there was nothing. In two and a half months, her brain was, as far as the MRI could tell, free of cancer. On April 21, a PET scan was performed, and it showed the same wonderful void—there was no metabolically active tumor to be seen.

As spring turned into summer, Marianne had regained a bit of her former strength but was still weak. The routine of her life had returned, and things began to fall back into a version of normalcy. Her awful diagnosis seemed more like part of someone else's life, a fading nightmare. Another MRI was scheduled for July 22. This one would reveal if the cancer, beaten back by the treatment, had come out of hiding. Like the previous scans, the MRI showed that her cancer was still nowhere to be seen. Marianne decided that it was time to relax the austere diet she had done for seven months. The process had sapped her strength, and she felt that she had little left to fight with. She stopped R-KD after her MRI on July 22.

On October 9, less than three months after stopping R-KD, Marianne was scheduled for another MRI, and this time, it was bad news. Her cancer was back. "The results didn't ignite fear or anxiety— she only felt sad to be leaving her family," Zuccoli said, "She knew what loss was, her father was taken by the Nazis when she was three years old." She knew that a reoccurrence of glioblastoma came with no hope.

They discussed her options. She could try the diet again if she wanted to, but it was too much. She had no energy left to fight.

"Probably she was no longer motivated to fight. Probably she had already decided to leave. She felt that her condition was very stressful upon her family," Zuccoli said. He prescribed her Avastin, a decision that he said he regretted. "Now we know that Avastin does not prolong survival. It does modify the appearance of the tumor, but rather than stopping the tumor's growth, it causes it to grow in infiltrative patterns," he said. But the chemotherapy had little effect on Marianne's cancer, and it took her life in a few months.

The fact that the return of the cancer coincided directly with the loosening of the diet might have been coincidence, or it might not. Even though the trial consisted of a single patient, it produced an amazing result. Prior to this study, Seyfried and others could find no reports showing regression of a glioblastoma within two and a half months using standard treatment alone. This suggested that the diet strongly impacted the tumor by cutting off its only source of energy. Marianne's glioblastoma, one of the hardiest, grittiest cancers to treat, was dissolved and untangled from her neuronal network, but as compelling as the result was, it would have to be proven in a larger trial.

By 2010, with the results of the Wurzburg trial, Nebeling's trial, and Seyfried's case study known, restricted, therapeutic ketosis appeared to be a viable approach against cancer. How well it worked, the types of cancer it worked best on, and how to fine-tune it were questions that remained to be answered. Only large clinical trials would answer them. As Seyfried's lab continued its frenzied quest to discover methods to exploit cancer metabolically, it saw a theme emerging. The trials so far gave researchers every reason to think that R-KD could stand alone therapeutically, but it was increasingly apparent that the diet's true power was in combination. When combined with other treatments, it prepped the therapeutic landscape in a spectacular way. Like an amplifier boosting the output of a stereo, the diet appeared to boost the efficacy of a variety of other therapies. It also appeared to condition normal, healthy cells to resist the toxic side effects of traditional cancer treatments.

The dual nature of the diet was backed by a series of studies. One study showed how the duality was achieved from the genetic level. Normal cells, battle hardened through eons of adaptation, swiftly orchestrated the genetic shift to ketone metabolism by tooling up the enzymatic machinery needed for the dietary transition. Unable to make the transition to ketosis, cancer cells were put under tremendous pressure, as the fuel they craved was replaced by one that they couldn't consume. The missing and damaged mitochondria, Seyfried reasoned, was the Achilles' heel of cancer cells. It left them metabolically hamstrung. His lab zeroed in on this weakness, bombarding the cell from every metabolic angle and capitalizing on its inflexibility.

Veech worked out a biochemical map showing how entering ketosis translated into a differentiation between normal cells and cancer cells. The ketogenic diet, as he showed, supercharged normal cells, lifting them to a vigorous state of health. In addition to bathing the cells in a superefficient fuel, ketone bodies do something else: they prepare normal cells to deal with free radicals—the hyperactive wrecking balls blamed for every malady from cancer and neurodegeneration to the mother of all disease: aging itself. A close look at the labels in any grocery store highlighted the threat of free radicals—food companies packed food full of antioxidants and advertised them boldly on the packaging.

Antioxidants are the antithesis of free radicals because of their ability to neutralize them. Beyond the antioxidants people consumed, their cells manufacture an antioxidant called glutathione that is responsible for neutralizing the bulk of the free radical assult. Glutathione is so important to the "good side" of the oxidative battle (that has been waged since the days of the primordial ooze) that researchers dubbed it the "master antioxidant." As Veech noticed, ketone bodies dramatically tilted the ratio of armed glutathione (the antioxidant form) to unarmed glutathione, beefing up the cellular defense of healthy cells as they transitioned to ketone body metabolism. As healthy as the conversion to ketosis was for normal cells, it was equally and inversely detrimental to cancer cells, widening the therapeutic gap alluded to earlier. Unable to make the transition, cancer cells had to rely on a different pathway to arm glutathione—a pathway that relied on glucose. As the transition to ketosis drove down blood glucose, a cancer cell had both its energy source and its capacity to prepare glutathione for battle against free radical assault taken away.

For a cancer patient, R-KD made healthy cells healthier and cancer cells sicker. This prepped the therapeutic landscape for other therapies, making them more effective and less toxic.

The Most Important Game in Town

R-KD's ability to prep the therapeutic landscape is not trivial. It achieves a unique therapeutic duality, preparing normal cells to withstand oxidative assault while simultaneously making cancer cells more vulnerable to it. In fact, from a therapeutic point of view, the interplay between free radicals and antioxidants may be the most important game in town. Watson has certainly come to believe so. His 2012 manifesto, the work he claimed "was his most important since the double helix," was titled "Oxidants, Antioxidants and the Current Incurability of Metastatic Cancers," a title highlighting the new-found importance he placed on the dueling pair. The bulk of the article was devoted to sorting out the relationship between free radical-inducing therapies and antioxidants within cancer cells, the importance of which, Watson said, is vastly underappreciated.

This relationship is important for two reasons. First, the most important pathway to kill cancer cells is through apoptosis, and it appears that apoptosis in many cases is triggered by quick bursts of free radicals. Second, many current cancer therapies operate by inducing bursts of free radicals, thus triggering apoptosis.

Free radicals are also called reactive oxygen species (ROS), and research has shown that cancer cells have unusually high amounts of ROS. Most ROS is generated as a byproduct of mitochondria metabolism, so the damaged mitochondria in cancer cells are likely to "leak" much more ROS, leaving cancer cells in a precarious state of oxidative chaos. Watson said that many more cancer therapies than previously thought probably work by nudging cancer cells over the oxidative edge by overloading them with ROS. He contends that entire classes of chemotherapeutic drugs in all probability operate by generating an intolerable amount of ROS, killing the cancer cell in the process. The "first in class" mitochondrial drug elesclomol, developed by Synta Pharmaceuticals, killed by promoting ROS generation. Proof that elesclomol operates through ROS generation is easy to come by. Simply coaxing the cell to manufacture more of the antioxidant glutathione halts the drug's "preferential killing of cancer cells," Watson wrote.

To Watson, this epiphany was his most important since his discovery of DNA: "All these seemingly unrelated facts finally make sense by postulating that not only does ionizing radiation produce apoptosis through ROS but also today's most effective anti-cancer chemotherapeutic agents."

But Watson's sudden epiphany came with a catch-22. If he was right, the antioxidants that researchers said were making us healthy would make most forms of chemotherapy less effectual. In fact, he noted, antioxidants could even help to cause cancer in the first place. The paradox inspired him to write, "In light of the recent data strongly hinting that much of late-stage cancer's incurability may arise from its possession of too many antioxidants, the time has come to seriously ask whether antioxidant use much more likely causes than prevents cancer." Could it be that the antioxidants people were told were nutritional saviors were *causing* cancer? There was evidence to back up Watson's statement. At the least, researchers could say with confidence that, with respect to cancer, antioxidants had the potential to rescue cancer cells from the very therapies that doctors were using to kill them.

The importance of the paradox merged seamlessly with the metabolic approach to cancer therapy. The delivery of ROS as a death sentence for cancer cells fit with the biochemical mechanism of Seyfried's R-KD, which, in theory and supported by evidence, suggested that we could have our cake and eat it too. Rather than the possibility that antioxidants might diffuse into cancer cells through the blood stream and thwart the ROS needed to induce apoptosis, R-KD did the opposite. It cut off the cancer cell's ability to manufacture its most important antioxidant—glutathione—rendering it defenseless against most cancer treatments. As an added bonus, because R-KD affected cancer cells and normal cells differently, the diet forced healthy cells to manufacture more glutathione, thus preparing them for the corrosive effects that ROS-generating therapies collaterally imposed on healthy tissue. R-KD appears as a dream scenario: it sensitizes cancer cells to ROS, leaving them perched on the edge of a cliff, while it prepared the rest of the body to handle any additional ROS-generating therapies, thus minimizing side effects.

Two questions required experimental evidence to prove the dual nature of the diet. First, by prepping normal cells to handle ROS, did R-KD attenuate the side effects, promoting tolerability of ROS-generating therapies? And second, did R-KD *enhance* ROS-generating therapies like radiation? Experimental evidence strongly suggests that the answer to both questions is yes.

Valter Longo of the University of Southern California, an Italian-born researcher, is passionately interested in how diet affects cancer and aging in general. Longo is a rising star in the field of aging research, and like Seyfried, his research led him to cancer. To answer the first question, Longo tried to convince oncologists to have patients with a variety of cancer types fast before, during, and after chemotherapy sessions. Fasting is essentially the same as R-KD, it is the quickest route to ketosis. He came up with his own name for the therapeutic duality achieved by ketosis: differential stress resistance (DSR).

Longo set out to test whether fasting could curb the well-known side effects of chemotherapy, but he ran into friction while trying to recruit patients. Even though he explained to oncologists that fasting results in DSR and should greatly improve the outcome of their patients and mitigate side effects, they were dubious. He wrote, "As expected, many clinicians were skeptical of our hypothesis that cancer treatment could be improved not by a 'magic bullet' but by a 'not so magic DSR shield.'" The skepticism was highlighted by Leonard Saltz, an oncologist at Memorial Sloan Kettering Cancer Center. When asked about enrolling patients in Longo's trial, Saltz said, "Would I be enthusiastic about enrolling my patients in a trial where they're asked not to eat for two and a half days? No."

Eventually Longo convinced ten oncologists to allow their patients, suffering from malignancies ranging from stage 2 breast cancer to stage 4 esophageal, prostate, and lung malignancies, to undergo a prechemotherapy (48–140 hours) and a postchemotherapy (5–56 hours) water-only fast. Across the board, the fasting patients reported less severe side effects in fourteen different categories. Subjective side effects like fatigue, nausea, headaches, weakness, memory loss, numbness, decreased sensation, and tingling were all reported as less severe as were measurable effects like vomiting, hair loss, diarrhea, and mouth sores. The trial provided empirical evidence that fasting prepared normal cells to withstand a chemotherapeutic assault.

The second question: does fasting or R-KD sensitize cancer cells, rendering them more susceptible to ROS-generating chemotherapies? Several lines of evidence suggested that the answer is yes. A group headed by Adrienne C. Scheck at the Barrow Neurological Institute in Arizona showed that R-KD alone slowed the growth of tumors in mice, but when combined with radiation treatment, the result went from good to outstanding, with many of the mice achieving a full cure. This hinted at the reason for Marianne Zuccoli's remarkable regression from the diet combined with radiation.

Seyfried showed the synergy between the diet and a drug called 2-deoxyglucose (2DG), a molecule that looked like glucose but could not be further metabolized, effectively bringing fermentation to a halt. The diet or the drug alone showed the ability to slow tumors, but when combined, Seyfried found that the result was profoundly synergistic.

Longo then showed that mice with brain cancer experienced extended survival when they fasted before the administration of temozolomide and radiation. It seemed that in every scenario, entering ketosis enhanced other therapies while keeping toxic shrapnel from damaging healthy tissues. The diet appeared to slow cancer growth, but that alone did not appear to be R-KD's strong suit. The way it prepared the therapeutic landscape made it unique. It was like primer to a painter or fertilizer to a gardener. It conditioned the environment in which the cancer existed, enhancing other therapies while attenuating side effects.

Gorgeous in Concept (More of the Same)

In 2011, the FDA approved the drug ipilimumab for the treatment of late-stage melanoma. It was one of the first of a new class of targeted immunological cancer drugs, a class with hopes so high that *Science* magazine labeled the emerging therapies the "breakthrough of the year" for 2013. To apply the word "breakthrough" after years of marginal if not outright failed attempts to treat late-stage melanoma implied that the drugs must have had a meaningful impact.

The theory behind the drugs was gorgeous in concept. They operated by harnessing the latent power of the immune system. Rather than stimulate the immune system, ipilimumab worked by uninhibiting a class of cancer-killing immune cells called cytotoxic T lymphocytes (T cells), unleashing the aggressive mercenary cells and allowing them to patrol the body without caution. For those suffering from late-stage melanoma, ipilimumab equated to an increased survival of four months on average, but uninhibiting cytotoxic T-cells comes with a price. Ipilimumab acts by cutting the brake lines on aggressive immune cells. Sometimes the cells reach their targeted destination, and other times, they end up crashing into a bystander. In addition to endocrine disruption, stomach pain, diarrhea, fever, breathing and urinating problems comes a risk of outright death. In a trial of 540 patients, three saw their cancer melt away, but fourteen were killed, giving patients a risk of death five times greater than cure. This high-stakes game of Russian roulette comes at a price of $120,000 per treatment of four infusions over three months.

Press-Pulse

When you see Dominic D'Agostino, you don't think scientist. The University of South Florida professor has a passion for nutrition and fitness, and in a charity fundraiser, he broke the Guinness World Record for the most weight squatted in twenty-four hours (175,500 pounds in less than six hours, breaking the old record by more than 50,000 pounds).

Mitochondria: An Old Theory Is New Again

Like Seyfried, D'Agostino is a virtual encyclopedia of knowledge on the subject of cancer metabolism, and like good scientists everywhere, he didn't set out to study the metabolism of cancer but was led to it by observation. "The last thing I wanted to do was study cancer. It seemed like a lot a people studying it just couldn't get a handle on it," he said.

After finishing his PhD, he received a grant from the Office of Naval Research to study the cellular and molecular effects of oxygen toxicity, which is a limitation to Navy SEAL divers using closed-circuit breathing apparatus. To do this D'Agostino's team built a creative tool. They placed an atomic force microscope inside of a hyperbaric oxygen chamber, allowing them to see in real time the effects oxygen pressure had on different cell types. The experimental tool was a hit. D'Agostino and his students excitedly documented the effects of increased oxygen pressure on different types of cells. One particular cell type caught D'Agostino's attention. The cells appeared particularly vulnerable to the damaging effects of high concentrations of oxygen. "The cells were bubbling up and then exploding," he said. "I didn't even know where this immortalized cell line originated." When he investigated the origin of the cells he discovered that "they were glioblastoma cells from a 44 year old stage-four cancer patient."

The observation sent his career on a new trajectory. He had already delved deeply into nutritional ketosis as a way to mitigate seizures and other side effects that SEALs might experience from oxygen toxicity. He knew the diet protected neurons from a variety of insults, so it was easy to connect the dots. "We did an experiment that showed ketones could kill cancer cells by themselves," he said. The swirling observations led him to Seyfried's 2010 journal article, *Cancer as a Metabolic Disease*. The comprehensive theory Seyfried laid out tied everything D'Agostino had seen firsthand into a unified whole.

Seyfried was in Boston working on R-KD, noticing how it proved synergistic with ROS-generating therapies, while D'Agostino was observing the ROS-generating ability of hyperbaric oxygen chambers to explode cancer cells. In addition to saturating pockets of tissue that may be hypoxic, hyperbaric oxygen generates ROS, the crucial element of most cancer therapies (according to Watson). A phone call was all it took. Seyfried and D'Agostino recognized the potential and worked out a collaboration.

The experiment they designed was simple. In a highly metastatic mouse model of brain cancer, they measured the effect of R-KD plus hyperbaric oxygen. The results, published in the summer of 2013, gave testimony to the power of the simple union. By themselves, R-KD and hyperbaric oxygen slowed tumor growth, but together, they eviscerated it. The diet alone increased mean survival by 56.7 percent compared to the control mice, and when it was combined with hyperbaric oxygen, the mean survival jumped to 77.9 percent.

Because they believe in the metabolic theory of cancer, Seyfried and D'Agostino approach cancer therapy from a different angle. Their vision is almost utopian—a therapeutic approach less like combat and more like a gentle rehabilitation and restoration of health. They envision treating patients with a "synergistic combination of nutritional ketosis, cancer metabolic drugs (like 3BP, DCA, and 2DG) and hyperbaric oxygen therapy (HBOT)." Their vision is not a bombardment based on the "no pain, no gain" mentality that the early pioneers, DeVita and Pinkel employed. They liken it to a "press-pulse" scenario similar to the ecological phenomenon known to cause mass extinctions. Their description of cancer as an "ecosystem" is an honest image of the complex nature of the disease. Cancer *is* an ecosystem, rife with interwoven relationships and Darwinian selection pressures. As any ecologist would tell you, the best way to alter an ecosystem is to change the entire environment rather than targeting an isolated variable. That is the approach D'Agostino and Seyfried envision. They focus on changing the entire environment in which the cancer tries to live.

The diet gently "presses" on the cancer, weakening it and rendering it vulnerable. Metabolic therapies then provide the "pulse," pushing the weakened cells over the edge. They term the overall approach "mitochondria enhancement therapy."

For the cancer cell, R-KD with HBOT turns a windless, sunny day into a hurricane with driving wind, pelting sheets of rain, and flooding streets. It is easy to get excited by their vision. "Can you imagine coming out of chemotherapy healthier than you came in? That's the way it should be! The process should be a restoration!" Seyfried said. Even though they are quick to temper expectations, when Seyfried and D'Agostino speak, it is easy to detect the confidence they have in their approach and their excitement at the implications. It is possible that one day R-KD combined with HBOT could replace radiation altogether, especially considering that HBOT is able to target cancer anywhere in the body and radiation is not. They say that R-KD combined with HBOT "could potentially kill tumor cells as effectively as radiation without causing toxic collateral-damage to normal cells."

Are Seyfried and D'Agostino right? Is R-KD with HBOT as or more effective than standard radiation therapy, and could it be proven beyond a shadow of a doubt in clinical trials? If so, the world would be presented with a much better option, one that improved the health of the patient as the therapy was administered over time. An additional caveat is that the therapy is dirt cheap when compared to radiation. It would be a turning point and a massive step in the direction of cheap, nontoxic, effective health care. For the most lucrative branch of medicine, radiation oncology, it would mean "pink slips" on an unprecedented scale throughout cancer centers all over the world. It is not unrealistic to expect friction.

The same is true for 3BP. If 3BP lives up to its promised ability to treat a multitude of cancer types, it would revolutionize cancer treatment. Like R-KD with HBOT, it appears to be a largely nontoxic therapy that could potentially treat any cancer that was PET positive, which equates to 95 percent of cancers. Rather than treat cancer as two hundred different diseases, 3BP and R-KD with HBOT treat cancer as one disease. The amount of 3BP that eradicated Yvar's cancer cost less than $100. R-KD was essentially free, although a cancer center would have to retrain staff nutritionists, and HBOT was comparatively cheap. In Seyfried and D'Agostino's vision, a cancer center would be a clinic where patients went to restore or "enhance" their damaged mitochondria and, in a nontoxic and orderly manner, kill off the diseased cells. There would be no buckets to throw up in and no bald patients with lifeless expressions, shells of their former selves. There would be no medical bankruptcies or families scrambling to pay for drugs that cost more than $100,000 for a single treatment course that was of almost no benefit. There would be no radiation burns or subversion of healthy cells to cancerous ones cast forth by the treatment itself, no massive increase in acquiring cancer later in life from dripping war gas into people's veins.

When cancer is framed as a metabolic disease, the entire paradigm of treatment is turned inside out. Doctors are treating a single disease, and they are treating "sick" cells, not the immortal, super cells that the genetic theory paints them as. Was this vision realistic? The treatments are in their infancy—this is the first act in treating cancer as a metabolic disease. Only time will tell.

The preclinical experiments, case studies, and trials that have been done exhibit incredible promise as do the anecdotal stories that the span the country. The problem is money. Because metabolic cancer treatment is so cheap, ironically, it is difficult to get funding. Something seems off when a drug like Herceptin, that treats only a fraction of one type of cancer and is of marginal benefit, rallied the likes of patient advocacy groups all the way to Hollywood and big corporate money, while therapies like R-KD, HBOT, and 3BP, therapies that have the potential to help so many, sit on the sidelines. Why aren't people demanding that these therapies be pushed through clinics?

Abrahams has firsthand experience with trying to get an incredibly effective, free dietary therapy for pediatric epilepsy established in hospitals. "Ironically, the biggest obstacle we have is the fact that the diet is free," he said.

Part 7

Where Do We Go from Here?

Siddhartha Mukherjee's *The Emperor of All Maladies* is a rich and exhaustive narrative, a true biography of cancer. The vast account begins with a question: is the end of cancer conceivable? Is it possible to eradicate this disease from our bodies and societies forever?

The question is more relevant than ever. Cancer is on the march and will soon pass heart disease as our number one killer. As Mukherjee explains, "Indeed the fraction of those affected by cancer creeps inexorably in some nations from one in four to one in three to one in two, cancer will, indeed, be the new normal—an inevitability." In 2014, the World Health Organization issued a report warning of an upcoming "tidal wave" of cancer, reporting that fourteen million people are diagnosed with cancer each year. That is predicted to increase to nineteen million by 2025, twenty-two million by 2030, and twenty-four million by 2035.

Can cancer be defeated? Mukherjee's conclusion is grim, casting the disease into something inexorably knitted into the fabric of our existence. He writes,

Where Do We Go from Here?

Cancer is stitched into our own genomes...We can rid ourselves of cancer, then, only as much as we can rid ourselves of the process in our physiology that depends on growth—aging, regeneration, healing, reproduction...It is unclear whether an intervention that discriminates between malignant and normal growth is even possible.

A victory over cancer, he says, "would be a victory over our own inevitability—a victory over our own genomes."

Like the majority of cancer researchers today, Mukherjee believes that cancer is purely genetic—born out of random mutations that will inevitably occur within our DNA, so intertwined with our thread of life that it is impossible to untangle—an interpretation that leads to a cul-de-sac of untreatable inevitability. But his conclusion is based on an *interpretation* of the science describing the nature of cancer. Cancer is only cast as an inevitability, *if*, in its heart of hearts, it is caused and driven by mutations to DNA. The answer to this question depends on the nature of the beast—a scientific detective story that is still unfolding.

It is a strange time for the basic biology of cancer. TCGA was supposed to be our final battle—all roads led to it. At no time in history have we had such exquisite tools to view cancer. In the past, scientists tried to piece together a complex murder mystery using a crackling, old radio that cut out for extended periods only to briefly turn on and provide glimpses of the story. Today, at least with respect to genetic mutations, scientists view the story in high definition from beginning to end. And it has shown cancer to be a disease of biblical complexity—causing many to pause—forcing cancer's preeminent researcher, Vogelstein, to fill the void of understanding with something not yet discovered, an ephemeral "dark matter," an elegant way of saying "we don't know." At the same time, emerging evidence cast the metabolic theory into a new light, thrusting its viability far past Warburg's single observation.

I use James Watson's story as a common thread through this book for many reasons—partly because he discovered DNA, the molecule thought to be the center of cancer, and partly because of his iconic status in the cancer research community, but mostly because of his thinking on the direction that cancer research should go: away from genetics and toward metabolism and ROS therapies. I wish I had been able to interview him or at least thank him, but my attempts went unanswered. I don't know what he would have said about 3BP and if his interpretation of events is different from Pedersen's or Ko's. But it is clear from his writings that he recognizes the tremendous potential of the molecule.

Most scientists are convinced that cancer was established as a genetic disease decades ago. This view appears now to have been one dimensional, and it ignores evidence that looks at cancer in two or three intertwined dimensions. Some scientists are coming around to the idea that cancer might be a metabolic disease—not because anybody convinced them to think differently, but because the science led them there. The position that cancer is caused solely by mutations to key genes is becoming harder to maintain. The inconsistencies are too numerous and pronounced. No researcher today can point to any single mutation or any combination of mutations and say with confidence that it alone is the cause of cancer. Nor can researchers point to a series of cellular systems rendered dysfunctional by mutations and make the same claim with confidence.

Cancer is perceived as a predictable manifestation of a universe that tends toward chaos—that favors disorder over order—it is seen as accidental. Although the origin of cancer may be the result of chaos the disease itself is anything but. It takes a remarkable amount of coordination to do what cancer does, to go through the elaborate functionality of the cell cycle flawlessly and repeatedly. To transition to energy creation by fermentation means that the cell must drastically alter its enzymatic profile in an orderly manner. To direct the growth of new vessels to feed the growing mass takes an exquisitely complex series of operations. Cancer is a disease of order, and at every step of the way, it is directed and coordinated from somewhere.

There was a poignant difference in feeling from scientists who espoused the SMT compared to those who championed the metabolic theory. The genetic camp felt almost defeated, like a dead end had been reached. There was an undeniable aura of loss and "where do we go from here?" In sharp contrast, the scientists who back the metabolic theory of cancer—Seyfried, Pedersen, D'Agostino, Ko, and others—exude excitement. Their labs bubble like Silicon Valley start-ups. They feel that they are on to something big. When I ask most scientists about the inconsistencies embedded in the genetic theory, I'd usually get a quizzical look followed by the statement, "Well, cancer is more complex than we thought." Most do not question the SMT and are largely unaware of the profound inconsistencies that plague the theory.

When Varmus and Bishop discovered that the RSV contained a slightly distorted version of one of our own genes, it seemed like a trick. Could a virus really capture a single gene and reinsert its malevolent doppelganger directly into DNA, resulting in a disease characterized by complexity? Deleting some amino acids from a single kinase protein results in a disease that can grow new blood vessels to supply its needs and undergo the remarkable biochemical shift to glucose metabolism, all due to a few missing amino acids? The process seems unlikely.

Rous never believed in the SMT of cancer and vehemently argued against it. But Varmus and Bishop made Rous appear the fool when they showed that the virus that bore his name had committed treason by incontrovertibly confirming the SMT. "Nature has a sardonic sense of humor," Rous said of cancer's deck of trick cards. Was he wrong? When it was proven that the Rous virus concentrated its pathology within the mitochondria, a new question emerged. What was transforming the cell: the single, altered protein product of the Rous viral src gene or a distress call from badly damaged mitochondria to a plethora of signaling hubs, activating a coordinated response and manifesting the complex operations of the cancer cell? One was a single mutation; one of an almost infinite combination that seemingly could manifest in the same disease. The other, a process active in every cancer cell regardless of tissue type, as PET scans allude to.

If time proves that the metabolism of cancer is more important than previously thought—maybe the precipitating or "big bang" event we have been desperately chasing—then, as Rous suggested, nature will have deceived us again. Whether God, Mother Nature, evolution, or whatever shaped the world we live in, we must concede that in the realm of disease, cancer is her masterpiece. It is the Bobby Fischer, the George Patton, the Mozart, the Houdini, and the Einstein of maladies. The way she has enticed us with understanding only to pull it out of our reach is horrible and, I dare say, even beautiful. Cancer is pathological artistry. Even Sherlock Holmes respected the master criminal he could not catch.

Could we have mischaracterized the true nature of cancer? If so, Mother Nature shoulders the burden of blame. With exquisite deception, she covered one theory with the other, artfully tangling them so that one looks like the other. She put some diseases into tidy categories, displaying the underling mechanism that causes them plainly for us to see, but not with cancer. It contains cover ups, trip wires, deceptions, and false leads. It is the puzzle of all puzzles. History is replete with examples of brilliant men and women getting the answers to large questions wrong, even though they followed the evidence and drew conclusions based on what they knew at the time. Throughout history, great scientists have been victims of circumstance.

Where Do We Go from Here?

Look no further than Rous, who appeared dead wrong in his assertion that cancer was not caused by mutations to DNA. Had he lived long enough, he might have been vindicated. Theories rise and fall. They are ephemeral, fleeting entities that morph as we view Mother Nature from different angles. They dance and pirouette as they travel their circuitous path through time. They make some look the fool while turning others into heroes. All good scientists must agree that timing, circumstance, and blind luck play a huge role in the destiny of a career and how history will judge their work. Had Watson and Crick dragged their feet while attempting to elucidate the structure of DNA, their Nobel Prize might have been snapped up by American scientist Linus Pauling (who was also building models in his lab and was close to determining DNA's structure). Had Pauling been slightly faster, nobody might know the names Watson and Crick today. Seyfried admits as much: "Ten years from now, some scientist might prove that I was completely wrong." He's right. The continuum of science has little room for ego.

This is not a standoff between one theory and another. Nature is under no obligation to present cancer as a genetic disease or a metabolic disease exclusively. It may be that the SMT of cancer and the metabolic theory are intertwined—a chimerical monster, existing in two realms at once. Nature still doesn't have to make the answer easy. As the metabolic theory is reborn from the ashes, its overlap with the SMT appears like a setup. Rather than existing in sharp contrast, the theories are one shade off. They hide each other and cover for each other, like mischievous kids gleefully enjoying the deception.

If some diseases are single frames, cancer is a full-length feature film. Through the iterative process of science, investigators have been able to capture still shots of the movie to examine in two dimensions. Even with TCGA filling in a large gap, we have yet to view the film from beginning to end. Scientists have to guess what's in the gaps.

They have to theorize what the entire movie will look like. Einstein used thought experiments to work out the problems of physics. At the age of sixteen, for hours, or even days on end, Einstein would imagine the laws of physics as he toured the universe riding on a beam of light. From that unique perspective he was able to map out the basic principles of relativity. I can't help but imagine what it would be like to be able to witness the movie of cancer from beginning to end. To be able to sit there and watch as all the gaps are filled in.

Whatever the exact nature of cancer is, the metabolic and genetic theories propose vastly different therapeutic scenarios. Warburg, Pedersen, Ko, Seyfried, D'Agostino, and others invoke an image of cancer that isn't painted on a tapestry of inevitability. They view cancer as a disease with a single, understandable flaw. The metabolic theory illuminates the disadvantage of cancer and exposes its Achilles' heel. Cancer cells are not immortal, gritty, adaptable supercells. That is the description of healthy cells that have evolved through millennia of harsh conditions. Seyfried once said, pointing to a slide showing normal cells, "These cells have earned the right to be on the planet!" Pointing to cancer cells, he said, "These cells have not!" The healthy cells in our bodies are the resolute survivors. They live through and bounce back from the toxic sludge that is most chemotherapy, while many of the cancer cells die off. Healthy cells can transition to accommodate ketosis, while cancer cells are left sputtering in their inflexibility.

We have not been at this very long at all. The first chemotherapy was developed in the middle of World War II. By letting highly toxic substances flow through the veins of patients, cancer cells are preferentially (to a small degree) killed off, highlighting that they are more vulnerable than healthy cells. If scientists have mischaracterized the origin of cancer, then we have lost three decades trying to target mutations that are a side effect rather than the motor driving the disease.

Where Do We Go from Here?

If cancer is metabolic, we are just getting started, and real progress should be quick to follow. We will find more ways to push the sick cells over the edge.

What will the future of cancer treatment be? The SMT of cancer tells us that cancer is fatally conjoined to us. It tells us that to defeat cancer, we must target an infinitely complex enemy that is always evolving and perpetually one step ahead. Researchers must develop a vast armament of targeted drugs to treat hundreds of different driver mutations. Experience tells us that to target the founder series of mutations that supposedly precipitate the malignancy, sometimes is not enough. It tells us that intratumoral heterogeneity is a therapeutic checkmate. At distant sites even within the original tumor, other drivers will develop, and they must be targeted too. If a doctor is lucky enough to have a drug for that new mutation, then he and his patient are one step ahead in the battle. But off in a microscopic corner, a new driver develops. In time it will smolder into its own, and it must also be sequenced and targeted. It is a perpetual game of "catch me if you can." Therapy would consist of sequencing followed by chemo, followed by sequencing, trying to chase down the enemy. And this assumes that driver mutations are initiating and perpetuating the disease at all.

If Warburg was right, and cancer originates from injured respiration, therapeutic strategy and drug design have to be completely reconfigured. Rather than attacking a hazy, morphing target that by its nature cannot be directly hit, researchers will be presented with a single target that permeates the spectrum of disease. This implies that cancer cells are not mutated versions of cells with superpowers programmed by an omniscient supervillain. They are damaged cells trying to survive in their own misguided way. They can be corralled, guided, manipulated, and killed.

The metabolic therapies highlighted here are the first attempts of a few scientists to combat cancer from a new perspective. For a first attempt, they give much reason for hope. They offer a sharp departure from the past. Cancer therapy could be a gentle rehabilitation. Like Seyfried says, "You should come out on the other side healthier than when you came in."

The scientist has a duty to temper expectations until clinical trials unequivocally prove efficacy. They are quick to say, "We have to wait and see." But before GLEEVEC went into clinical trials, it was supported by a single publication, summarizing five simple experiments in mice and petri dishes suggesting that it might work in humans. Three BP is far past that. It has shown stunning results in animals that surprise veteran cancer researchers, *and* it has demonstrated a relentless ability to wipe out cancer in a human case study. It was tied up in a squabble, but that is over. All Dr. Ko needs to launch 3BP into a small trial is about $3 million. Trials for R-KD combined with HBOT also need about $3 million.

The beautiful thing about R-KD with HBOT is that it could be used as an adjunctive therapy because it is nontoxic. It could also be put to work when conventional treatment is over and patients are sent home into a suspended purgatory. Their questions lingering: "Is my cancer still there? Is it growing back?" R-KD with HBOT would keep them in the fight during this uncomfortable phase. But the combination therapy of R-KD with HBOT might even prove better than most others, including radiation, giving patients a much better and affordable nontoxic option. In Seyfried and D'Agostino's "press-pulse" vision, treatment would be a rehabilitation where R-KD with HBOT were combined with other treatments (perhaps 3BP, DCA, and other drugs known to target metabolism). It could be administered continuously unlike conventional chemotherapy that has to be frequently halted due to anemia, low white blood cell counts, renal failure, liver toxicity, and nerve damage. Researchers need support to get these therapies into clinical trials. It would take one major benefactor to prove the efficacy of these treatments, maybe offering humanity a better, more affordable form of medicine.

Cancer is still climbing. It is still becoming more and more of a burden to our friends, neighbors, and the people we love. Some leading scientists have publicly announced that they are moving on from TCGA—there is nothing else to learn. Perhaps it is time for NCI to focus on the metabolic theory of cancer. Even if we've tripped over the truth while trying to discover the nature of cancer, it's not too late. Repeating the nuclear transfer experiments might be a good place to start. Cancer biology could learn from physics: "Get to the heart of the theory, and stop worrying about the periphery." We must illuminate Vogelstein's dark matter if we are to understand cancer and develop treatments. And the metabolic theory might be the best place to start looking.

If you would like to help realize the potential of metabolic therapies go to: SingleCauseSingleCure.org

Appendix A

Putting Metabolic Therapies to Work

The way the R-KD works is simple. Cancer needs glucose to survive. When glucose is restricted, the cancer cell is forced to compete with healthy cells for any available glucose. And while healthy cells effortlessly transition to burning ketone bodies, cancer cells, unable to, are put under tremendous metabolic and oxidative pressure. It is simple, elegant, and rational.

According to Seyfried and D'Agostino the foundation of metabolic therapy begins with the restricted ketogenic diet. It "presses" on cancer cells metabolically, weakening them, making them more vulnerable. Preclinically, and in case studies, the diet has been shown to slow tumor growth. In addition the diet sets the stage, as we've discussed, for additional treatments. In preclinical models the diet has been shown to be synergistic with a variety of other cancer treatments, enhancing their outcome while minimizing the toxic collateral damage that comes with many standard treatments.

Appendix A

Implementing the Restricted Ketogenic Diet

Of course anyone who wants to try the R-KD should only do it under the supervision of a healthcare provider. If your doctor is unfamiliar with the diet, there are others who can help. See Appendix B.

The best way to start the diet is with a water-only fast for 48 to 72 hours. This is also what doctors recommend for seizure patients. It is the fastest way to enter ketosis. First the patient must be determined to be in good enough health to undergo a fast. Some may chose to begin gradually. This may be done by simply starting the maintenance phase of the diet.

The diet itself is pretty simple. First, reduce your carbohydrate intake to less than 12 grams per day. Second, eat only .8 to 1.2 grams per kg of body weight per day of quality protein. And finally, the rest of the diet consists only of fat. But make sure it is the good variety, like olive oil, coconut oil, and butter from grass-fed cows, for example.

There is no one size fits all restricted ketogenic diet. It is a game of constant monitoring. The aim is to flip the ratio of glucose to ketone bodies. Normally a healthy person will have blood glucose under 100 mg/dl and no circulating ketone bodies. The goal is to drive blood glucose down to a steady level of approximately 70-80 mg/dl and blood ketones to 2 to 4 millimolar. Dr Seyfried calls this the "therapeutic zone"—a physiological state that is very hostile for cancer cells, yet very healthy for normal cells. Seyfried recommends checking blood glucose and ketones three times a day. Dr. D'Agostino recommends using the Medisense Precision Xtra blood glucose and ketone monitor (Abbott Laboratories) which you can buy at CVC or Walgreens. He found it easiest to use and the most accurate. Monitoring should be done before breakfast, and about two hours after lunch and dinner. Be sure to keep a log. That way you can learn which foods spike glucose and avoid them. Everyone has a unique metabolism so no two diets will be the same. The most important aspect of the diet is restriction. Even if a ketogenic diet is followed perfectly, too much of it will allow blood glucose to drift out of the zone. It is the restriction of overall calories that matters the most for the diet to work. While one patient might do fine on 1200 overall calories, another might only need 800. This can only be determined through constant monitoring.

Key points:

- If determined by your doctor to be safe, the best way to start the KD-R is by a 48 to 72 hour water only fast.
- Try to maintain a ratio of 4 grams of fat to every gram of protein, with total carbohydrates below 12 grams per day.
- Reduce overall calories until the therapeutic "zone" is reached.
- Monitor blood glucose and ketones up to three times a day.
- Remember, the most important part of the diet is overall caloric restriction.
- Only attempt the KD-R with a healthcare provider.
- *Remember, the most important part of the diet is overall caloric restriction.*

Dr. George Yu is a urological surgical oncologist and Professor at George Washington University Medical Center. For 13 years Dr. Yu has witnessed the power of merely restricting cancer patient's diets to 1200 – 1500 calories a day of nutrient dense food, free from sugars, fruits, and dairy. "Approximately one-third of the patients have impressive regressions, some even achieving complete remissions," says Dr. Yu, "The other two-thirds will improve but then they develop a recurrence and die. The diet slowed, but did not change the outcome. But it is clear, even in the most aggressive cases, *caloric restriction appears to slow tumor growth."* Dr. Yu's version of caloric restriction is different form Dr. Seyfried's, but he has nevertheless seen impressive results, pointing to the efficacy of overall caloric restriction. However, there are many reasons why the R-KD might be better than just restricting calories without worrying too much about the diet's composition. First, the R-KD is able to bring blood glucose lower. Second, because quality fats make up the majority of calories, ketones are more easily manufactured. And as we know, cancer cells have a reduced capacity to burn ketones, AND ketone bodies by themselves have been shown to be toxic to cancer cells. And finally, the high fat composition of the R-KD makes the caloric restriction more manageable, (less hunger) and therefore helps with compliance.

The idea of fasting or greatly restricting calories is counterintuitive for some. Dr. Seyfried highly recommends reading *Fasting for the Renewal of Life* by Herbert M. Shelton. The book helps to dispel any fears about caloric restriction, and highlights the many health benefits gained by caloric restriction. In this book, the great scientist Richard Veech touts the many benefits of ketosis. Human physiology was made to withstand caloric restriction. Veech is convinced many of our modern ills might be cured by simply eating less.

What can I eat? Great question. We will give you examples soon but there are many resources to help you. One of the best is the Charlie Foundation. The Charlie Foundation recently changed its name from "The Charlie Foundation for Pediatric Epilepsy" to "The Charlie Foundation for Ketogenic Therapies". The name change was inspired by a recent increase in requests for help using the diet for cancer and neurological disorders. "In the past most people wanted help with epilepsy, today half of the people who contact us are interested in using the diet for other purposes," said Jim Abrahams, founder of the Charlie Foundation. Their website contains an abundance of resources from food suggestions, to recipes, to current clinical trials studying the ketogenic diet's effect on cancer. (There are nine trials currently recruiting!)

Beth Zupec-Kania, the head nutritionist for the Charlie Foundation, below summarizes the basic dietary guidelines that she forged from working with many cancer patients.

Ketogenic Diet Therapy

Ketogenic diet therapy for cancer can be divided into two stages, an aggressive treatment phase and a maintenance plan. The aggressive phase starts with a fasting period and advances to a calorically controlled diet plan. This phase is maintained for several weeks and up to two months. The maintenance phase is meant to provide sufficient calories to maintain lean body weight. A nutrition therapist can formulate a diet plan for both phases including a prescriptive amount of fat, carbohydrate and protein to meet individual needs and specify supplements to prevent nutrient deficiencies.

Starting Ketogenic Therapy

Fasting is often used as a preparation for ketogenic therapy and can be helpful in depleting the rapid source of stored energy (called glycogen) and promoting ketosis. Once stored glycogen levels are near depletion, glucagon becomes elevated which stimulates fat breakdown to make ketones.

This change in metabolism may affect people differently. Individuals including young children, those who are underweight, and those who are receiving certain medications (especially those that cause acidosis), are at increased risk for adverse effects. Acidosis and dehydration are two effects that could result from fasting therefore medical supervision is advised. People with a fatty-acid metabolism disorder should not attempt ketogenic diets.

Appendix A

Fasting

Fasting includes eliminating all foods and beverages and consuming only water. Carbohydrate-free electrolyte water may be used to prevent loss of electrolytes particularly sodium and potassium and prevent acidosis. Sufficient fluid should be consumed to prevent dehydration; approximately 2 liters for an adult.

The length of the fast depends upon the results achieved during fasting including degree of weight loss and glucose levels. Fasting glucose levels between 60-80 mg/dL are typical for adults. The glucose range is typically 10 points lower for children and minimal to no fasting is needed to achieve this.

Starting The Diet

Since the ketogenic diet is highest in fat, gradual initiation to the full plan is often better tolerated. The small volume and fat-rich content of meals are best savored slowly. During the aggressive phase of diet therapy, just two meals daily with one or two high-fat snacks is sufficient for most adults (not for children). Ketosis diminishes appetite and reduces desire to overeat. The caloric level of the diet is based on body size, activity level, age and gender.

Monitoring

It is essential during fasting phase and during diet therapy to monitor blood glucose levels and ketones. Portable meters are available that can measure blood levels of both. High glucose levels can indicate excessive calories while low glucose levels can indicate insufficient calories. High glucose levels may also be present if too much protein is consumed. Similarly, high glucose levels in an individual who is underweight may indicate the breakdown of body protein which is not good. Weighing oneself every few days is another necessary monitor. The state of ketosis causes a diuretic effect resulting in weight loss from loss of body fluid which may be 5-10% of body weight. This is why it is imperative to hydrate with fluids.

Miriam Kalamian's Story

Another nutritionist with a great deal of experience implementing the restricted ketogenic diet for cancer patients is Miriam Kalamian. In the winter of 2004 Miriam's four year old son, Raffi, was diagnosed with a brain tumor. Three surgeries and as many failed chemotherapeutic regimens later they were told there was nothing left to do. With nothing to lose, Miriam discovered Dr. Seyfried's research and his unique dietary protocol. With the help of Raffi's pediatrician and oncologist they began the restricted ketogenic diet along with a low dose of chemotherapy (the same regimen that had failed to work earlier). Amazingly, the tumor shrank by 15% in the first 3 months! Chemo was discontinued in December of 2007 and Raffi continued with the ketogenic diet as his sole therapy for three more years. Miriam was stunned by the results, and amazed others were unaware of this powerful, non-toxic therapy, she has made it her life's work to help others with metabolic cancer therapy. You can read more about this in her latest ebook titled, *Get Started with the Ketogenic Diet for Cancer: A Step-by-Step Guide to Implementation.* Here is her brief summary of what can be eaten, and what should be avoided when using the KD-R for treating cancer.

The Ketogenic Diet For Cancer
Once you've determined that you're a good candidate for a ketogenic diet, it's time to set your plan in motion. First, purge your home of all foods that are not keto-friendly. This is true even if other family members are not adopting this same lifestyle. Let them go other places to

get their fix of foods not on your plan. Kids are especially adept at hiding low-quality foods so don't feel that you need to hold onto that bag of M&M's to keep life "normal" for their sake!

As you shop for keto-friendly foods, you'll be cruising new corners of your supermarket or natural foods store. Focus on fresh or frozen foods. You don't need to be a gourmet cook to prepare a healthy and satisfying meal! If this concept is new to you, start simple. Go online to look for a few keto-friendly options that look interesting then set out to gather the ingredients you'll need. At the same time, pick up any special kitchen equipment that will ease preparation (such as a silicon spatula or wire whisk).

Let's Start With What You Can Have! What follows is NOT a complete list- instead; it's a place to start. Use the info on the following pages to prepare a shopping list. Choose foods that you already enjoy but also be sure to try one or two new foods each week. You're sure to find a few new favorites!

Vegetables
The emphasis here should be on *non-starchy* choices. When possible, choose organically raised foods.

- Asparagus
- Broccoli
- Brussels Sprouts
- Cabbage
- Cauliflower
- Celery
- Cucumbers
- Greens (for sautéing)
- Kale
- Mushrooms

- Salad Greens
- Spinach
- Zucchini

After you are keto-adapted, you can add back in limited amounts of these foods:

- Garlic
- Onions
- Peppers
- Tomatoes

Fruits

Despite what you hear about the antioxidant properties of fruit, our bodies are not adapted to handling a high intake of fructose (a.k.a., "fruit sugar"). This is even more problematic for people with cancer. Fruits raise blood glucose/insulin and interfere with keto-adaptation. Wait until you're keto-adapted before adding limited amounts of certain low-sugar berries or fruit back into your diet. Even then, always combine them with fats to lower their impact on blood glucose levels.

- Apple- a few (4-5) very thin slices
- Berries- such as blackberries, raspberries, or strawberries (blueberries are higher in sugars)
- Grapefruit- a few sections
- Test the effect of your fruit choices by using a home blood glucose monitor

Proteins

Whenever possible, choose meats from pasture raised or "free range" animals. These have a healthier fat profile than animals that are fed grains. "Organic" is a bonus. Although most animal proteins contain no carbohydrate, carbs from eggs and shellfish should be counted as part of your daily intake. Note that even "uncured" bacon and sausage usually contains nitrates "naturally occurring in celery juice" (or beet powder).

- Beef
- Lamb
- Pork (including limited amounts of bacon and sausage)
- Poultry
- Seafood (wild caught fish and shellfish)
- Wild game meats
- Eggs (look for those that are high in omega-3's)

Dairy

Milk is not keto-friendly as it is high in lactose ("milk sugar"). Other dairy products can be classified as either high FAT or high PROTEIN. High FAT dairy (cream, butter) contains estrogen metabolites that may be problematic for people with hormone-sensitive cancers. High PROTEIN dairy (cheese, yogurt) can stimulate insulin production as well as provide a source of IGF-1, which can accelerate growth of most tumor tissue. Limit dairy intake and choose products from animals that have been pasture raised. "Organic" is a bonus. Most dairy contains some carbohydrate- count it as part of your daily intake.

- Butter, clarified butter, or ghee (mostly fat but still considered "dairy")
- Cheese ("hard" cheeses such as cheddar or Parmesan OR soft high-fat cheese such as Brie)
- Heavy whipping cream

- Cream cheese
- Sour cream (cultured, without added starches or fillers)
- Yogurt- IF you want to include yogurt, use plain full-fat unsweetened yogurt with no starchy fillers or additives- strain the liquid and only use small amounts of the solids)

Nuts And Oils

For now, keep to this "short list" of keto-friendly nuts and seeds. Also, consider limiting your intake to 2 oz. or less per day as most contain high levels of pro-inflammatory omega-6 fatty acids. All nuts contain some carb and protein. Research your favorites to evaluate the pros and cons of each.

- Almonds
- Brazil nuts
- Coconut meat- unsweetened
- Hazelnuts
- Macadamias (good choice- highest in fat; lowest in carbs and protein)
- Pecans
- Walnuts (good choice- fewer omega-6's than most nuts)
- Chia seeds
- Flaxseeds (rich in healthy omega-3's and fiber- grind and store in the refrigerator)
- Hemp hearts/seeds

Avocados And Olives

These two foods deserve a special mention. Both are high in healthy monounsaturated fats. Both can also help to boost the fat content of a meal. For example, ½ of an average Haas avocado provides 2 tsp (approximately 10 g)of fat with little carb or protein. One caveat: if you are allergic or sensitive to latex, you may also have a cross reaction to certain foods. Avocado is near the top of that list.

- Avocados -Haas (mainly from Mexico or California- smaller than the Florida variety)
- Olives (use more like a condiment)

Fats And Oils

Keto diets are very high in fat so quality, composition, and "balance" is important. Look for cold-pressed organic varieties and limit your intake of "refined" (solvent-treated) oils. Never use soy or vegetable oils- they are very high in omega-6's. When using oil for sautéing, use the lowest heat possible. Take the time to learn more about fats, oils, and cooking methods. (I include a comprehensive section on fats in my eBook.)

- Animal fats and lard
- Butter or ghee (if dairy is included in the diet)
- Coconut oil and MCT oil derived from coconut oil- balance your intake
- Omega-3 fish oils, either as fresh fish (e.g., wild caught salmon) or in purified supplements
- Olive oil (extra virgin for dressings; extra light for cooking)
- Salad dressings and mayonnaise- preferably homemade using olive oil
- "Buttery Spreads" such as Earth Balance- preferably organic
- Other oils based on personal preferences (e.g., flaxseed, almond, avocado, macadamia)

Sweeteners

I consider it essential that you lower your "sweet thermostat". This will aid in compliance as it reduces the seductive hard-wiring in your brain that can result in a sweets binge. Dulling your desire for sweets may also protect against an inadvertent rise in insulin that can accompany the simple *thought* of eating sweet foods.

- Stevia- liquid drops
- Erythritol- small amounts, such as what's found in Truvia
- Splenda in very limited amounts ONLY until you transition to stevia or no sweetener at all!

Spices, Flavorings, And Seasonings

These items add variety and interest to your meals. Some also have health benefits as anti-inflammatories or aid in maintaining blood glucose control.

- Basil, black pepper, cayenne pepper, chili pepper, chives, cilantro, coriander seeds, cinnamon, cloves, cumin seeds, curry, dill, ginger, mustard seeds and prepared mustard, nutmeg, oregano, paprika, parsley, peppermint, rosemary, sage, thyme, and turmeric. (These are suggestions, NOT a complete list)
- Curry, garlic powder, and onion powder (count the carbs)
- Salt- any variety. Most people on a ketogenic diet need to add salt to foods or broths
- Traditional condiments- check labels for sugars and carbs
- Lemon juice- up to one tablespoon per day
- Vinegar- distilled or apple cider is best- no balsamic or malt
- Pure extracts, such as vanilla. orange oil, or peppermint- limit to a few drops
- Sugar-free foods, such as pancake syrup- use sparingly as they often contain poor quality ingredients
- Be careful with commercial spice mixes- they often have added sugars or starches so read ingredient labels carefully

- Avoid ANY seasoning that lists monosodium glutamate (MSG) or any type of hydrolyzed vegetable/soy protein as these may be especially harmful for individuals with cancer
- Unsweetened cocoa powder deserves some mention here but use it sparingly

Baking Soda And Baking Powder

Both of these are keto-friendly and commonly used in baking. Baking POWDER contains some carbohydrate (and possibly aluminum). Baking SODA (contains no aluminum) may reduce metastatic spread in certain cancers *when added to water and sipped between meals* (this may not be appropriate for everyone- look into the research on this).

- Baking SODA
- Baking POWDER

Beverages

This best liquid is water! The diet is slightly dehydrating so be sure to drink enough to replace what you lose throughout the day. Other beverages add variety. Avoid those with artificial sweeteners.

- Water
- Clear broth or bouillon
- Decaf coffee & tea
- Herbal tea (check the ingredients for flavorings that may add carbs)
- Seltzer water (zero carb), club soda, and limited amounts of stevia-sweetened drinks- read the labels to be sure that there are no unwanted ingredients, such as aspartame or sucralose
- Unsweetened almond or flax milk- these are low in carbs and great as a base for protein shakes

- Unsweetened boxed coconut milk "beverage"- this is NOT the canned coconut milk used in Asian cooking

  ★ Addicted to caffeine? Before you start the diet, cut back to ½-1 cup in the morning or eliminate it entirely. Caffeine may raise blood glucose and can also contribute to the dehydrating effect of the diet.

Meal Planning Is Crucial For Success!

This "template" can ease your transition to a ketogenic diet but there's more to meal planning than simply having the right foods on hand. You also need to determine how much of each type you'll need. Dealing with cancer has its own set of challenges, making this plan different from standard ketogenic diets for weight loss. I strongly recommend that you seek guidance from a nutritionist that specializes in ketogenic diet therapy to help you individualize your initial plan and troubleshoot issues that may arise, especially in the early weeks and months of the diet. Consider purchasing my eBook as one of your resources: <u>Get Started with the Ketogenic Diet for Cancer: A Step-by-Step Guide to Implementation</u>.

<u>Breakfast</u>

1. Pick your favorite (eggs? bacon? cheese? protein shake?)
2. What fats and oils will work with this meal? (butter? coconut oil? cream?)
3. Veggies (spinach? tomato?), berries, or <2 g carb bread/roll (almond? flax?)

Example: Egg Breakfast- 2 eggs with a strip of bacon (add butter to the beaten raw eggs) AND a serving of vegetables sautéed in olive oil OR ¼ cup berries with cream.

Lunch
1. Start with 2-3 cups of salad greens and/or ½ of an avocado
2. Add your protein food (Chicken? Tuna? Sardines?)
3. Serve with olive oil and/or salad dressing and/or mayo

Example: Chicken Caesar Salad- 2 cups of salad greens with ½ of an avocado and "deck of card" portion of cooked chicken. (You can reduce the chicken portion to allow for some grated parmesan.) Serve with olive oil dressing and any vinegar except balsamic

Dinner
1. Pick your protein first (Salmon? Chicken?)
2. Select veggies and other foods (Broccoli? Sesame seed?)
3. Choose a combo of complementary fats & oils (Butter? Olive oil? Mayo?)

Example: Fish Dinner: Baked or poached fish ("checkbook" sized) with a vegetable such as broccoli or asparagus (~ ½ - cup raw) sautéed in olive oil. Serve with mayo.

Add a Snack: 1 TBS almond butter with 2 tsp of coconut oil, spread on celery "boats".

If you are faced with challenges (extensive liver disease, GI compromise, poor nutritional status, low thyroid), **consider these changes to the basic meal plan:**

★ Add another serving of non-starchy vegetables and/or avocado
★ Keep oils at a level that does not induce nausea or vomiting
★ Split your meals (and your fats) into smaller portions

SAY "NO" TO THESE FOODS AND ADDITIVES!

- **NO SUGARS– read ingredient labels carefully!**
  No agave nectar, honey, molasses, and evaporated cane juice. Identify other sources of sugars by their "-ose" endings (sucrose, dextrose, maltose). Avoid sucralose as well. This is NOT a complete list. If in doubt, check the Internet. (Start by looking up "maltodextrin", an ingredient all too common in many packaged foods.)

- **NO GRAINS**
  No wheat, corn, oats, rye, barley, spelt, triticale, quinoa, bulgur, groats. It is increasingly clear that even people without cancer should eliminate or reduce their intake of grains.

- **NO STARCHY VEGETABLES**
  No potatoes, sweet potatoes, cooked carrots, beets, parsnips, yams, winter squash, peas.

- **NO STARCHY OR HIGH GLYCEMIC FRUITS**
  No bananas, citrus, pears, pineapple, or dried fruits of any kind. AFTER you are keto-adapted, small amounts of unsweetened berries (¼ cup) or a few very thin slices of apple may replace of a serving of vegetables once daily IF this doesn't cause a spike in glucose.

- **NO LEGUMES**
  No peanuts, soy, garbanzos, beans, dried peas, lentils. (Vegetarian or vegan plans generally need to include limited amounts of legumes to meet protein needs.)

- **NO MILK OR SOFT CHEESES- THEY CONTAIN CARBOHYDRATES (LACTOSE)**
  Fermentation and/or culturing may reduce lactose to keto-friendly levels but limit intake to strained solids. Cottage cheese is NOT recommended but if you do choose to include it, strain it! Limit intake from these sources to 2 tablespoons per day.

- **NO ALCOHOL (OR SUGAR ALCOHOLS) during keto initiation/adaptation**
  No foods with ingredients that ends in "-ol" (sorbitol, mannitol, maltitol). These interfere with ketosis. **Exception**: Small amounts of erythritol or xylitol may be OK with most people.

- **CITRATES SUPPLEMENTS CAN INTERFERE WITH KETOSIS**
  Limited amounts of citrates found in oral supplements (Vitamin C and certain magnesium supplements) are likely to be OK. Monitor your response. Intravenous Vitamin C MAY work synergistically with the diet in certain cancers. More research and clinical data are needed here.

As with any diet, compliance is the elephant in the room. Most people cheat on diets, and can convince themselves that "a little extra this or that won't hurt". When the ketogenic diet is used to repress seizures, the consequences of cheating are immediate, frightening, and obvious. However, when the R-KD is used for cancer the consequences are not immediate and obvious. Even worse, "getting off" sugar can be brutal. A lifetime of carbohydrate and sugar consumption mimics an addiction in every sense of the word. And with addiction comes withdrawn symptoms. Many feel intense cravings, lightheadedness, and irritability for a few days. But this will pass.

The "Pulse", the power of synergy

With the diet in place the foundation is set. The cancer cells are perched in the precarious state of energetic and oxidative stress. Now the hope is to apply "pulses" of stress that will push the cells into extinction. There is a lot of preclinical data, in both animals and humans, suggesting the R-KD will actually improve the outcome of *many* other chemotherapies, including radiation, while mitigating side-effects. The diet is the "press", while radiation and chemotherapy provide the "pulse." Additionally, Seyfried and D'Agostino showed that the R-KD combined with hyperbaric oxygen had extremely effective results in mice with highly invasive metastatic cancers. As hyperbaric oxygen is already approved for use to recover from the damage done by radiation therapy, doctors may be less hesitant to make the leap and suggest their patients also use it to attack cancer metabolically. If your doctor is unfamiliar with Seyfried and D'Agostino's study, the reference is below. As for other metabolic therapies, like DCA, and 3-Bromopyruvate, they are simply not yet approved for use. We hope that will change soon.

Poff AM, Ari C, Seyfried TN, D'Agostino DP: The ketogenic diet and hyperbaric oxygen therapy prolong survival in mice with systemic metastatic cancer. PLoS One 2013, 8:e65522.

Appendix B

List of known Doctors familiar with metabolic cancer therapies and might be willing to help:

Dr. Mark Renneker, UCSF (mark.renneker@ucsf.edu)

Dr. George Yu, George Washington Univ, Washington, DC (george. yu8@gmail.com)

Dr. Helen Gelhot, St. Louis, MO area (helengelhot@charter.net).

Dr. Simon Yu, St. Louis, MO (simonyumd@aol.com)

Dr. Greg Nigh, Portland, OR (drnigh@naturecuresclinic.com)

Dr. Robert Elliott, Baton Rouge, LA (relliott@eehbreastca.com)

Dr. Kara Fitzgerald, Hartford, CT (kf@drkarafitzgerald.com)

Dr. Ian Bier, Portsmouth, NH (ian@hnnhllc.com).

Dr. Neal Speight, North Carolina (nespeight@gmail.com)

Dr. Ouriana Stephanopoulos, Univ. Kansas, Kansas City (ostepha-nopoulos@kumc.edu)

The following nutritionists have a service for helping cancer patients implement the ketogenic diet. These nutritionists have in depth knowledge on how to implement the KD for cancer management.

Miriam Kalamian, EdM, MS, CNS   ((mkalamian@gmail.com). Miriam also has a new eBook entitled, *"Get Started with the Ketogenic Diet"*. The book is strongly recommended for those cancer patients who need help with ketogenic diet implementation and can be obtained from the following web site: (dietarytherapies.com).

Beth Zupec-Kania (ketogenicseminars@wi.rr.com).   Beth directs the Charlie Foundation, which focuses on the use of the ketogenic diet for epilepsy, and other diseases including cancer.

Ellen Davis has also prepared a short eBook that can help cancer patients implement the KD according to the ideas of Dr. Seyfried. Link to eBook purchase is here: http://www.ketogenic-diet-resource.com/cancer-diet.html

Notes

In The Beginning

Rome life expectancy: Frier, Bruce W. (2001). "More is worse: some observations on the population of the Roman empire". In Scheidel, Walter. Debating Roman Demography. Leiden: Brill. pp. 144–145

Life expectancy data: Galor, Oded & Moav, Omer (2007). "The Neolithic Revolution and Contemporary Variations in Life Expectancy". Brown University Working Paper. Retrieved 12 September 2010.

Health History hard Choices: Funding Dilemmas in a fast Changing World. University of Indiana. August 2006

CIA—The World Factbook—Rank Order—Life expectancy at birth

"Antibiotics": Surmise and Fact on the Nature of Cancer. Nature, May 16, 1959. Peyton Rous

"Artifact of civilization": Merchants of Immortality. Stephen Hall

CALICO: http://www.cnn.com/2013/10/03/tech/innovation/google-calico-aging-death/index.html

Cancer statistics: http://money.cnn.com/magazines/fortune/fortune_archive/2004/03/22/365076/index.htm

"cancer, above all other diseases": The Prime Cause and Prevention of Cancer, Otto Warburg, Lecture delivered to Nobel Laureates on June 30, 1966, at Lindau, Lake Constance, Germany

Marshall B: Helicobacter pylori: past, present and future. Keio J Med. 2003, 52(2):80-5.

"Barry J. Marshall - Biographical". Nobelprize.org. Nobel Media AB. 2013.

Marshall BJ: The pathogenesis of non-ulcer dyspepsia. Med. J. Aust. 143 (7): 319

"David Agus": http://caaspeakers.com/wp-content/uploads/2013/02/AgusD_CNNArticle.pdf

"The Cancer Genome Atlas": http://cancergenome.nih.gov/

"Article": http://robbwolf.com/2013/09/19/origin-cancer/

Otto Warburg: Cell Physiologist, Biochemist, and Eccentric. Hans Krebs, 1981 Clarendon Press Oxford.

"make no mistake" Vogelstein: interview with the author

Part 1: How Cancer Became a Genetic Disease

The Emperor of All Maladies, Siddhartha Mukherjee. I used Mukherjee's wonderful book as a resource to get the sequence of important events into a story like format. I indulged in some artistic license with Pott's walk into inner-city London, and "getting into the head" of Rous on his cattle drive, Warburg after his famous Lindau speech, and adding the pint of beer to the famous Eagle Pub event.

Chimney Boys

Life expectancy industrial revolution: Mabel C. Buer, Health, Wealth and Population in the Early Days of the Industrial Revolution, London: George Routledge & Sons, 1926, page 30

"Diseases in industrial cities in the Industrial Revolution". Historylearningsite.co.uk

http://ocp.hul.harvard.edu/contagion/tuberculosis.html

Pott's disease: Surgens-net. Percivile Pott

Waldron, H.A. A brief history of scrotal cancer. British Journal of Industrial Medicine 40 (4): 390–401 "a lodgement of soot in the rugae of the scrotum":http://www.whonamedit.com/doctor.cfm/1103.html

"Uncovering the cause of "phossy jaw" Circa 1858 to 1906: oral and maxillofacial surgery closed case files-case closed". J. Oral Maxillofac. Surg. 66 (11): 2356–63.

Chaotic Chromosomes

Virchow: Rines, George Edwin, ed. "Virchow, Rudolf". Encyclopedia Americana, 1920

David Paul von Hansemann: Contributions to Oncology: Context, Comments and Translations. Leon P. Bignold, Brian L. D. Coghlan, Hubertus P.A. Jersmann

Is Cancer Infectious?

Peyton Rous: http://www.nobelprize.org/nobel_prizes/medicine/laureates/1966/rous-bio.html

Rous P. A TRANSMISSIBLE AVIAN NEOPLASM. (SARCOMA OF THE COMMON FOWL.). J Exp Med. 1910, 12(5):696-705

Rous P. A SARCOMA OF THE FOWL TRANSMISSIBLE BY AN AGENT SEPARABLE FROM THE TUMOR CELLS. J Exp Med. 1911, 13(4):397-411

Notes

Warburg's War

Otto Warburg: Cell Physiologist, Biochemist, and Eccentric. Hans Krebs, 1981 Clarendon Press Oxford

Known carcinogens: US Department of Health and Human Services. Public Health Service, National Toxicology Program. Report on Carcinogens, Twelfth Edition. 2011. Accessed at http://ntp.niehs.nih.gov/ntp/roc/twelfth/roc12.pdf on June 14, 2011

Warburg O.: On respiratory impairment in cancer cells. Science 1956, 124(3215):269-70.

Warburg O.: On the origin of cancer cells. Science 1956, 123(3191):309-14.

"Even if Warburg is right": G. Lenthal Cheatle: An Address on THE PROBLEM OF CANCER. Br Med J. 1928, 2(3522): 1–4

Cancer. Am J Public Health Nations Health. 1930, (8):860-1.

Frank L. Horsfall, Jr. Current Concepts of Cancer. Can Med Assoc J. 1963, 89(24): 1224–1229

Voegtlin C.Present Status of Research in Cancer. Am J Public Health Nations Health. 1942, 32(9):1018-20.

Cramer W. The Origin of Cancer in Man in the Light of Experimental Cancer Research. Yale J Biol Med. 1941, (2):121-38

The Secret of Life

The Double Helix, James Watson

Frank L. Horsfall, Jr. Current Concepts of Cancer. Can Med Assoc J. 1963, 89(24): 1224–1229

A Question That Had Passed Him By

Otto Warburg: Cell Physiologist, Biochemist, and Eccentric. Hans Krebs, 1981 Clarendon Press Oxford.

Nature of Lindau meeting: http://www.lindau-nobel.org/The_ Mediatheque_Project.AxCMS?ActiveID=2373

Everything Was in a Fog

"I had an interest, I hate to admit it, in psychiatry" http://www.nobel-prize.org/mediaplayer/index.php?id=1682

"dangerously late in a prolonged adolescence": Ibid

"I knew from that moment, my life had changed": Ibid

"were really the only game in town": Ibid

"I soon learned how much more important a new measurement was than an old theory": Ibid

"It was like watching a puzzle solve itself": The Emperor of All Maladies, Siddhartha Mukherjee

Part 2: Chemotherapy and the Gates of Hell

The National World War II Museum. Early Cancer Treatment Discovered During the Aftermath of the Air Raid on Bari. Dec. 3, 2013

Ships sunk at Bali: http://www.warsailors.com/singleships/boll-sta.html

Contents of John Harvey: Coningham, Orange

Saunders, D.M.: "The Bari Incident". United States Naval Institute Proceedings (Annapolis: United States Naval Institute).

Lindskog: The Emperor of All Maladies, Siddhartha Mukherjee

"If one reads the literature at the time": A History of Cancer Chemotherapy, Vincent T. DeVita Jr., and Edward Chu

How Nitrogen Mustard works: Rink SM, Solomon MS, Taylor MJ, Rajur SB, McLaughlin LW, Hopkins PB (1993). "Covalent structure of a nitrogen mustard-induced DNA interstrand cross-link: An N7-to-N7 linkage of deoxyguanosine residues at the duplex sequence 5'-d(GNC)". Journal of the American Chemical Society 115 (7): 2551–7.

Side Effects of Nitrogen Mustard: http://chemocare.com/chemo-therapy/drug-info/Nitrogen-Mustard.aspx#.UysC9FPnbrc

Miller, DR. A tribute to Sidney Farber – the father of modern chemotherapy. British Journal of Haematology 134 (1): 20–26

Sidney Farber: The Emperor of All Maladies, Siddhartha Mukherjee

"Change the face of cancer drug development": A History of Cancer Chemotherapy, Vincent T. DeVita Jr., and Edward Chu

Marx, Vivien. 6-Mercaptopurine. Chemical & Engineering News. Retrieved October 20, 2012

Ying and Yang

2nd Reading from Making Cancer History - Frei and Freireich Combination Chemotherapy, M. D. Anderson Cancer Center

The ASOC POST, Emil 'Tom' Frei III, MD, Trailblazer in the Development of Combination Chemotharapy, Dies at 89, 5/6/2013

FREI E 3rd, HOLLAND JF, SCHNEIDERMAN MA, PINKEL D, SELKIRK G, FREIREICH EJ, SILVER RT, GOLD GL, REGELSON W.

A comparative study of two regimens of combination chemotherapy in acute leukemia. Blood. 1958, (12):1126-48.

Emil J. Freireich, Frei E 3rd. Confrontation, passion, and personalization. Clin Cancer Res. 1997, (12 Pt 2):2554-62

Freireich EJ, Karon M, Frei E III. Quadruple combination therapy (VAMP) for acute lymphocytic leukemia of childhood. Proc Am Assoc Cancer Res 1964; 5: 20.

"Volcanic": David and Goliath, Gladwell

"I'd never seen a ballet": Ibid

"Of the fourteen": Ibid

"These drugs do more harm than good": Ibid

MOPP

"Suddenly surrounded": ONI Sits Down with Dr. Vincent DeVita. 2008. http://www.cancernetwork.com/articles/oni-sits-down-dr-vincent-devita

"It took plan old courage": A History of Cancer Chemotherapy, Vincent T. DeVita Jr., and Edward Chu

DeVita VT, Serpick A. Combination chemotherapy in the treatment of advanced Hodgkin's disease. Proc Am Assoc Cancer Res 1967; 8: 13.

DeVita VT, Serpick AA, Carbone PP. Combination chemotherapy in the treatment of advanced Hodgkin's disease. Ann Intern Med 1970; 73: 881–95.

Notes

Total Therapy

"Each was raised by impoverished": Science Connections, Wilsede, Feb. 2008

"Never run from a fight": https://www.roswellpark.org/donaldpinkel

"Well this is it, I'm not going to wake up": Ibid

"I thought I was immune to it": Ibid

"By the end": A History of Cancer Chemotherapy, Vincent T. DeVita Jr., and Edward Chu

"eighty percent cured": Pinkel D. Treatment of childhood acute lymphocytic leukemia. Haematol Blood Transfus. 1979;23:25-33

"sixty percent cured from MOPP": A History of Cancer Chemotherapy, Vincent T. DeVita Jr., and Edward Chu

That Son of a Bitch

Nixons speech: https://www.youtube.com/watch?v=E2dzEDnGqHY

"Did we believe we were going to cure cancer": The Emperor of All Maladies, Siddhartha Mukherjee

"reprehensible": The Truth in Small Doses, Leaf

"The great naysayer of our time": Ibid

"referred to as that son of a bitch" Ibid

"We shall so poison": Robert Nisbet, Knowledge Dethroned: Only a Few Years Ago, Scientists and Intellectuals Had Suddenly Become the New Aristocracy: What Happened? New York Times, Sept. 28, 1975

"penicillin of cancer": http://cisplatin.org/

NCI drug screening factory: :A History of Cancer Chemotherapy, Vincent T. DeVita Jr., and Edward Chu "time and time again": http://www.nobelprize.org/mediaplayer/index.php?id=1542

Statistics: Treatment of Diseases and the War against Cancer. Scientific American 1985, 5(51-59)

Bailar JC 3rd, Smith EM. Progress against cancer? N Engl J Med. 1986; 314(19):1226-32

Survival data: Bhatia S, Robison L, Oberlin O., Greenberg M, Bunin G, Fossati-Bellani F, Meadows A, Breast Cancer and Other Second Neoplasms after Childhood Hodgkin's Disease. N Engl J Med 1996; 334:745-751

"Chemotherapy has, in fact," :A History of Cancer Chemotherapy, Vincent T. DeVita Jr., and Edward Chu

Part 3: Breakthroughs and Disappointments

Into the Dustbin of History

Otto Warburg: Cell Physiologist, Biochemist, and Eccentric. Hans Krebs

A Flickering Ember

Peter Pedersen, interview with the author

Pedersen PL: Tumor mitochondria and the bioenergetics of cancer cells. Prog Exp Tumor Res 1978, 22:190-274.

Bustamante E, Pedersen PL: High aerobic glycolysis of rat hepatoma cells in culture: role of mitochondrial hexokinase. Proc Natl Acad Sci U S A 1977, 74:3735-3739.

Bustamente E, Morris HP, Pedersen PL: Hexokinase: the direct link between mitochondrial and glycolytic reactions in rapidly growing cancer cells. Adv Exp Med Biol 1977, 92:363-380.

The PET Scan

Abass Alavi: interview with the author
   Peter Pedersen: interview with the author
   PET imaging: GE Healthcare

A New Era

HER 2, Robert Bazell
   "in the people magazine": Natural Obsessions, Natalie Angier
   "I don't like to owe": HER 2, Bazell
   "without Denny Slamon": HER 2, Bazell
   "the first step in the future": The Holtz Report, Herceptin: An Entirely New Weapon Against Cancer, Exclusive Report from the 1998 ASCO Meeting, Andrew Holtz http://holtzreport.com/SHNASCOHerceptin.htm
   Nobel Museum: Biography of Paul Ehrlich
   Herceptin survival statistics: "Ten Years Later, Trastuzumab Survival Advantages March On," Medscape, Neil Osterwell, December 07, 2012
   Hudis, CA (2007). "Trastuzumab--mechanism of action and use in clinical practice". N Engl J Med. 357 (1): 39–51.
   Herceptin Profit: http://www.gene.com/about-us/investors//historical-product-sales/herceptin

An Old Target is New Again

Young Ko and Peter Pedersen: interviews with the author

Apoptosis: Karam, Jose A. (2009). Apoptosis in Carcinogenesis and Chemotherapy. Netherlands: Springer.

Okouchi M1, Ekshyyan O, Maracine M, Aw TY: Neuronal apoptosis in neurodegeneration. Antioxidants & Redox Signaling2007, 9(8):1059-96.

"antisence RNA": DePalma, Angelo (August 2005). "Twenty-Five Years of Biotech Trends".

Case 1:05-cv-01475-WDQ In the United States District Court for the District of Maryland

Peter L. Pedersen: Warburg, me and Hexokinase 2: Multiple discoveries of key molecular events underlying one of cancers' most common phenotypes, the "Warburg Effect", i.e., elevated glycolysis in the presence of oxygen Journal of Bioenergetics and Biomembranes, 2007, 39(3) 211-222

Anastassios D. Retzios, Why Do So Many Phase 3 Clinical Trials Fail? Clinical R&D Services, 2009.

The Good, the Bad, and the Ugly

Young Ko, Peter Pedersen: interviews with the author

Case 1:05-cv-01475-WDQ In the United States District Court for the District of Maryland

I did not interview Dr. Dang or Dr. Watson and obtain their interpretation of events. All events came from the memory of Dr. Petersen, Dr. Ko, and the publicly filed court complaint.

If I Hadn't Seen it with My Own Eyes I Wouldn't of Believed it Harrie Verhoeven: interview with the author

Young Ko, Peter Pedersen: interview with the author
Email exchange: Dr. Vogl
Ko YH, Verhoeven HA, Lee MJ, Corbin DJ, Vogl TJ, Pedersen PL.: A translational study "case report" on the small molecule "energy blocker" 3-bromopyruvate (3BP) as a potent anticancer agent: from bench side to bedside. J Bioenerg Biomembr. 2012, 44(1):163-70
Farrah Faucett: http://www.dailymail.co.uk/tvshowbiz/article-1183415/Farrah-Fawcett-How-cancer-miracle-cure-turned-heartbreak.html

Cancer statistics: http://seer.cancer.gov/statfacts/html/all.html

Cancer statistics: http://www.cancer.org/cancer/leukemia-chronicmyeloidcml/detailedguide/leukemia-chronic-myeloid-myelogenous-key-statistics

Part 4: Dark Matter

"It has become axiomatic": http://www.nobelprize.org/mediaplayer/index.php?id=1542

Bush's speech on embryonic stem cells: http://news.monstersand-critics.com/northamerica/article_1094282.php

The Second Creation, Wilmut, Cambell, Trudge. Headline Book Publishing 2000

"We are close to transferring": Merchants of Immortality, Hall

"We are all born young": Ibid

Imputes behind Human Genome Project: http://www.normale-sup.org/~adanchin/populus/hgp.html

Info on Human Genome Project: http://www.genome.gov/10001772

"Grant incite": http://www.nytimes.com/1987/12/13/magazine/the-genome-project.html

"Biggest costliest": http://www.nytimes.com/1987/12/13/magazine/the-genome-project.html

Clinton's speech on the Human Genome Project: http://www.genome.gov/10001356

"We would not want one individual": http://articles.latimes.com/2012/jul/20/news/la-heb-myriad-breast-cancer-gene-james-watson-20120720

Cost to sequence genome: A Genome Deluge By ANDREW POLLACK Published: December 1, 2011, New York Times

TCGA annocment: http://cancergenome.nih.gov/newsevents/newsannouncements/news_12_13_2005

Is it Possible to Make Sense Out of This Complexity?

Bert Vogelstein: interview with the author

Getting to know Vogelstein: http://www.achievement.org/autodoc/page/vog0int-1

Vogelstein: http://www.hhmi.org/scientists/bert-vogelstein

Breakthrough Prize: http://articles.baltimoresun.com/2013-02-21/health/bs-hs-vogelstein-breakthrough-prize-2-20130220_1_cancer-research-hopkins-researcher-bert-vogelstein

What researcher were expecting to see, Emperor of all Maladies, Mukherjee. Also Vogelstein, interview with author.

Salk JJ, Fox EJ, Loeb LA: Mutational heterogeneity in human cancers: origin and consequences. Annu Rev Pathol 2010, 5:51-75.

Sjoblom T, Jones S, Wood LD, Parsons DW, Lin J, Barber TD, Mandelker D, Leary RJ, Ptak J, Silliman N, et al: The consensus coding sequences of human breast and colorectal cancers. Science 2006, 314:268-274.

Wood LD, Parsons DW, Jones S, Lin J, Sjoblom T, Leary RJ, Shen D, Boca SM, Barber T, Ptak J, et al: The genomic landscapes of human breast and colorectal cancers. Science 2007, 318:1108-1113.

Jones S, Zhang X, Parsons DW, Lin JC, Leary RJ, Angenendt P, Mankoo P, Carter H, Kamiyama H, Jimeno A, et al: Core signaling pathways in human pancreatic cancers revealed by global genomic analyses. Science 2008, 321:1801-1806.

A Paradigm Shift

"ad hoc": Soto A, SonnenscheParadoxes C,: Carcinogenesis: There Is Light at the End of That Tunnel! Disrupt Sci Technol 2013, 3:154-156

Jones S, Zhang X, Parsons DW, Lin JC, Leary RJ, Angenendt P, Mankoo P, Carter H, Kamiyama H, Jimeno A, et al: Core signaling pathways in human pancreatic cancers revealed by global genomic analyses. Science 2008, 321:1801-1806.

Parsons DW, Jones S, Zhang X, Lin JC, Leary RJ, Angenendt P, Mankoo P, Carter H, Siu IM, Gallia GL, et al: An integrated genomic analysis of human glioblastoma multiforme. Science 2008, 321:1807-1812.

Comprehensive molecular portraits of human breast tumours. Nature 2012, 490:61-70.

Salk JJ, Fox EJ, Loeb LA: Mutational heterogeneity in human cancers: origin and consequences. Annu Rev Pathol 2010, 5:51-75.

"bank tellers": Seyfried, Cancer as a Metabolic Disease

"There are enormous numbers of mutations present in each tumor": Loeb, interview with the author

Vogelstein B, Papadopoulos N, Velculescu VE, Zhou S, Diaz LA, Jr., Kinzler KW: Cancer genome landscapes. Science 2013, 339:1546-1558

"a typical metastatic lesion": 86 Vogelstein B, Papadopoulos N, Velculescu VE, Zhou S, Diaz LA, Jr., Kinzler KW: Cancer genome landscapes. Science 2013, 339:1546-1558

Charles Swanton: interview with the author

Notes

Rosalie Fisher, James Larkin, Charles Swanton: Inter and Intratumour Heterogeneity: A Barrier to Individualized Medical Therapy in Renal Cell Carcinoma? Front Oncol. 2012, 2: 49. Published online 2012 May 18

Charles Swanton: Intratumour Heterogeneity: Evolution through Space and Time. Cancer Res. 2012, 72(19): 4875–4882

The Turtle and the Rabbit

"isocitrate dehydrogenase": Parsons DW, Jones S, Zhang X, Lin JC, Leary RJ, Angenendt P, Mankoo P, Carter H, Siu IM, Gallia GL, et al: An integrated genomic analysis of human glioblastoma multiforme. Science 2008, 321:1807-1812.

"metformin": http://www.healthyfellow.com/308/metformin-and-cancer/

Wang Z, Lai ST, Xie L, Zhao JD, Ma NY, Zhu J, Ren ZG, Jiang GL. Metformin is associated with reduced risk of pancreatic cancer in patients with type 2 diabetes mellitus: A systematic review and meta-analysis.Diabetes Res Clin Pract. 2014 Apr 18. pii: S0168-8227(14)00190-9

"The reason the metabolism": Bert Vogelstein, interview with the author

Weinburg Hawaii trip: The Emperor of All Maladies, Siddhartha Mukherjee

Hanahan D, Weinberg RA: The hallmarks of cancer. Cell 2000, 100:57-70.

Metastatic mutations: 86 Vogelstein B, Papadopoulos N, Velculescu VE, Zhou S, Diaz LA, Jr., Kinzler KW: Cancer genome landscapes. Science 2013, 339:1546-1558

http://www.sciencedaily.com/releases/2011/03/110316113057.htm

Pedersen's talk: http://videocast.nih.gov/summary.asp?live=7542

Hanahan D, Weinberg RA: Hallmarks of cancer: the next generation. Cell 2011, 144:646-674.

Part 5: Watson Reconsiders

To Fight Cancer, Know the Enemy, James Watson, August 5, 2009, New York Times

Watson J, Oxidants, Antioxidants, and the current incurability of metastatic cancer. Open Biol. Jan 2013, 3: 120144

"Although no doubt unwelcome": http://www.redorbit.com/news/health/1112761440/dna-discoverer-james-watson-criticizes-cancer-research-011013/

Dr. Agus: http://caaspeakers.com/wp-content/uploads/2013/02/AgusD_CNNArticle.pdf

Experts question the benefit of high-cost cancer care, Medscape today, 2011

"If you can shrink the tumor": http://apricot-kernels.blogspot.com/2011/09/ralph-moss-on-chemotherapy-laetrile.html

Time to Consider Cost in Evaluating Cancer Drugs in United States? Medscape, 2009

"Vogelstein had moved on": interview with the author

Part 6: Mitochondria: An Old Theory is New Again

Mitochondrial theory of Aging: http://hplusmagazine.com/2011/10/21/the-mitochondrial-theory-of-aging/

Notes

"Life took over by networking": Sagan, Dorion; Margulis, Lynn (1986), Origins of sex: three billion years of genetic recombination, New Haven, Conn: Yale University Press

Mitochonria: http://lpi.oregonstate.edu/f-w00/aging.html

Mitochondria: http://www.sciencedaily.com/releases/2010/05/100525094906.htm

The Man who invented the Chromosome: a Life of Cyril Darlington Oren Solomon Harman (Harvard University Press, 2004)

"Darlington": Cancer as a Metabolic Disease, Seyfried

"Src has never conclusively": Alvarez RH, Kantarjian HM, Cortes JE, The role of Src in solid and hematologic malignancies: development of new-generation Src inhibitors. Cancer. 2006, 107(8):1918-29

Thomas Seyfreid: interview with the author

Erol A. Retrograde regulation due to mitochondrial dysfunction may be an important mechanism for carcinogenesis. Med Hypotheses. 2005;65: 525– 9.

Woodson JD, Chory J. Coordination of gene expression between organellar and nuclear genomes. Nat Rev Genet. 2008;9: 383– 95.

Chandra D, Singh KK. Genetic insights into OXPHOS defect and its role in cancer. Biochim Biophys Acta. 2010;1807: 620– 5.

The Society of Cells: Cancer Control of Cell Proliferation, Carlos Sonnenschein and Ana Soto

"Genes that respond": Cancer as a Metabolic Disease, Seyfried

"Anedocal cases": Dominic D'Agnostino, Thomas Seyfried, interview with the author

"Epigenetic just don't lend themselves": Vogelstein: interview with the author

Wallace D, The epigenome and the mitochondrion: bioenergetics and the evironment. Genes Dev. 2010, 24(15): 1571–1573

Israel BA, Schaeffer WI: Cytoplasmic suppression of malignancy. In Vitro Cell Dev Biol 1987, 23:627-632.

Shay JW, Werbin H: Cytoplasmic suppression of tumorigenicity in reconstructed mouse cells. Cancer Res 1988, 48:830-833.

Israel BA, Schaeffer WI: Cytoplasmic mediation of malignancy. In Vitro Cell Dev Biol 1988, 24:487-490.

"My only thought then": Schaeffer interview with the author

Shay, interview with the author

"And the beauty": Seyfried, interview with the author

"It is worth noting" Killing multiple myeloma cells with the small molecule 3-bromopyruvate: implications from therapy

Cancer as a Metabolic Disease, Seyfried

Wallace D, The epigenome and the mitochondrion: bioenergetics and the evironment. Genes Dev. 2010, 24(15): 1571–1573

Things May Not be as They Seem

The Emperor of All Maladies, Siddhartha Mukherjee

The Truth in Small Doses, Leaf

The New Era in Cancer Research, Varmus, Science magazine

"BCR-ABL found in normal people": Bose S, Deininger M, Gora-Tybor J, Goldman JM, Melo JV: The presence of typical and atypical BCR-ABL fusion genes in leukocytes of normal individuals: biologic significance and implications for the assessment of minimal residual disease. Blood 1998, 92(9):3362-7.

"Germline mutations": Cancer as a Metabolic Disease

"P53": Read, A. P.; Strachan, T.. Human molecular genetics 2. New York: Wiley; 1999. Chapter 18: Cancer Genetics

Varley J.M. "Germline TP53 mutations and Li-Fraumeni syndrome". 2003, Hum. Mutat. 21 (3): 313–20

"How p53, BRAC1, retinoblastoma, xeroderma pigmentosum, paraganglioma, and some forms of renal cell carcinoma could result in cancer through metabolic pathways": Cancer as a Metabolic Disease, Seyfried

Superfuel

"Fasting": Hippocrates, On the Sacred Disease, ch. 18; vol. 6

Wheless JW: History and origin of the ketogenic diet. Epilepsy and the ketogenic diet. Humana Press; 2004

Zupec-Kania BA, Spellman E: An overview of the ketogenic diet for pediatric epilepsy. Nutr Clin Pract. 2008, 23(6):589–96

"It was a fate worse than death": Charlie Abrahams, interview with the author

"Once I heard about the ketogenic diet": Charlie Abrahams, interview with the author

Veech R, Ketoacids? Good medicine? Trans Am Clin Climatol Assoc. 2003, 114: 149–163.

Veech RL, Chance B, Kashiwaya Y, Lardy HA, Cahill GF, Jr.: Ketone bodies, potential therapeutic uses. IUBMB Life 2001, 51:241-247.

"superfuel" Taubs, What if is all been a big fat lie, New York Times, 2002

Biochemistry of Ketosis: Veech, email exchange with author

Gasior M, Rogawski MA, Hartman AL: Neuroprotective and dis-ease-modifying effects of the ketogenic diet. Behav Pharmacol 2006, 17:431-439

Paoli A, Rubini A, Volek JS, Grimaldi KA.: Beyond weight loss: a review of the therapeutic uses of very-low-carbohydrate (ketogenic) diets. Eur J Clin Nutr. 2013 Aug;67(8):789-96.

Veech, R.L., The therapeutic implications of ketone bodies: the effects of ketone bodies in pathological conditions: ketosis, ketogenic diet, redox states, insulin resistance, and mitochondrial metabolism. Prostaglandins Leukot Essent Fatty Acids, 2004. 70(3): p. 309-19.

Neal, E.G., et al., The ketogenic diet for the treatment of childhood epilepsy: a randomised controlled trial. Lancet Neurol, 2008. 7(6): p. 500-6.

Henderson, S.T., et al., Study of the ketogenic agent AC-1202 in mild to moderate Alzheimer's disease: a randomized, double-blind, placebo-controlled, multicenter trial. Nutr Metab (Lond), 2009. 6: p. 31.

Siva, N., Can ketogenic diet slow progression of ALS? Lancet Neurol, 2006. 5(6): p. 476.

Maalouf, M., J.M. Rho, and M.P. Mattson, The neuroprotective properties of calorie restriction, the ketogenic diet, and ketone bodies. Brain Res Rev, 2009. 59(2): p. 293-315.

Stafstrom, C.E. and J.M. Rho, The ketogenic diet as a treatment paradigm for diverse neurological disorders. Front Pharmacol, 2012. 3: p. 59.

Hu, Z.G., et al., The protective effect of the ketogenic diet on traumatic brain injury-induced cell death in juvenile rats. Brain Inj, 2009. 23(5): p. 459-65.

Hu, Z.G., et al., Ketogenic diet reduces cytochrome c release and cellular apoptosis following traumatic brain injury in juvenile rats. Ann Clin Lab Sci, 2009. 39(1): p. 76-83.

Vanitallie, T.B., et al., Treatment of Parkinson disease with diet-induced hyperketonemia: a feasibility study. Neurology, 2005. 64(4): p. 728-30.

"The survival benefit is obvious": http://www.phschool.com/science/science_news/articles/ketones_to_the_rescue.html

P Rous, THE INFLUENCE OF DIET ON TRANSPLANTED AND SPONTANEOUS MOUSE TUMORS. J Exp Med. Nov 1, 1914; 20(5): 433–451

Otto Warburg: Cell Physiologist, Biochemist, and Eccentric. Hans Krebs, 1981 Clarendon Press Oxford.

Nebeling, Interview with the author.

Seyfried, Cancer as a Metabolic Disease

Seyfried, Interview with the author

Skinner R, Trujillo A, Ma X, Beierle EA: Ketone bodies inhibit the viability of human neuroblastoma cells. J Pediatr Surg 2009, 44:212-216; discussion 216.

Nemesis

T Seyfried, Zuccoli, Metabolic management of glioblastoma multiforme using standard therapy together with a restricted ketogenic diet: Case Report. Nutr Metab (Lond). 2010; 7: 33

Zuccoli, email exchange with the author

Veech R, Ketoacids? Good medicine? Trans Am Clin Climatol Assoc. 2003, 114: 149–163.

Veech RL, Chance B, Kashiwaya Y, Lardy HA, Cahill GF, Jr.: Ketone bodies, potential therapeutic uses. IUBMB Life 2001, 51:241-247.

Stafford, P., et al., The ketogenic diet reverses gene expression patterns and reduces reactive oxygen species levels when used as an adjuvant therapy for glioma. Nutr Metab (Lond), 2010. 7: p. 74.

The Most Important Game in Town

Watson J: Oxidants, antioxidants and the current incurability of metastatic cancers. Open Biol 2013, 3:120144.

Abdelwahab MG, Fenton KE, Preul MC, Rho JM, Lynch A, Stafford P, Scheck AC: The ketogenic diet is an effective adjuvant to radiation therapy for the treatment of malignant glioma. PLoS One 2012, 7:e36197.

Aykin-Burns N, Ahmad IM, Zhu Y, Oberley LW, Spitz DR: Increased levels of superoxide and H_2O_2 mediate the differential susceptibility of cancer cells versus normal cells to glucose deprivation. Biochem J 2009, 418:29-37.

Trachootham D, Alexandre J, Huang P. Targeting cancer cells by ROS-mediated mechanisms: a radical therapeutic approach? Nat Rev Drug Discov. 2009;8: 579– 91.

Lizzia Raffaghello, Fernando Safdie, Giovanna Bianchi, Tanya Dorff, Luigi Fontana, Valter D Longo Fasting and differential chemotherapy protection in patients. Cell Cycle. 2010 November 15; 9(22): 4474–4476

Marsh J, Mukherjee P, Seyfried TN: Drug/diet synergy for managing malignant astrocytoma in mice: 2-deoxy-D-glucose and the restricted ketogenic diet. Nutr Metab (Lond) 2008, 5:33.

Stafford, P., et al., The ketogenic diet reverses gene expression patterns and reduces reactive oxygen species levels when used as an adjuvant therapy for glioma. Nutr Metab (Lond), 2010. 7: p. 74.

Raffaghello, L., et al., Fasting and differential chemotherapy protection in patients. Cell Cycle, 2010. 9(22): p. 4474-6.

Zuccoli, G., et al., Metabolic management of glioblastoma multiforme using standard therapy together with a restricted ketogenic diet: Case Report. Nutr Metab (Lond), 2010. 7: p. 33.

Gorgeous in Concept (More of the Same)

Seyfried, Cancer as a Metabolic Disease

Couzin-Frankel J. Immune therapy steps up the attack. Science. 2010. 330: 440-3.

Press Pulse

D'Agnostino, interview with the author

Poff AM, Ari C, Seyfried TN, D'Agostino DP: The ketogenic diet and hyperbaric oxygen therapy prolong survival in mice with systemic metastatic cancer. PLoS One 2013, 8:e65522.

Seyfried TN, Flores RE, Poff AM, D'Agostino DP: Cancer as a metabolic disease: implications for novel therapeutics. Carcinogenesis 2014, 35:515-527.

"You should come out healthier" Seyfreid, interview with the author.

Part 7: Where Do We Go From Here?

The Emperor of All Maladies, Siddhartha Mukherjee

WHO Cancer Statistics: http://live.wsj.com/video/who-warns-of-tidal-wave-of-cancer/00B6831E-8D99-4CD0-9166-7FF8DD-B7A09B.html?mod=WSJ_article_outbrain&obref=obnetwork#!00B68 31E-8D99-4CD0-9166-7FF8DDB7A09B

"sardonic sense of humor": Rous P. The challenge to man of the neoplastic cell. Cancer Res. 1967, (11):1919-24

"vehemently argued": Rous P. Surmise and fact on the nature of cancer. Nature. 1959, 183(4672):1357-61

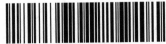

Made in the USA
San Bernardino, CA
28 September 2016